Strongheart

Strongheart

THE POWER TO
CONTROL DIABETES

A NOVEL BY

TERRI WOOD JERKINS

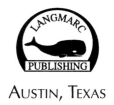

AUSTIN, TEXAS

Strongheart
THE POWER TO CONTROL DIABETES
BY TERRI WOOD JERKINS

Cover by Jeremy Jerkins

Copyright 2003 © Terri Wood Jerkins

Permission is granted by
Novartis Pharmaceuticals Corporation
to reference the Starlix™ name.

Permission is granted by
GlaxoSmithKline Pharmaceuticals
to reference the Avandia™ name.

First Printing 2004
Printed in the United States of America

Published by
LangMarc Publishing
P.O. 90488
Austin, Texas 78709-0488
www.langmarc.com

ISBN: 1-880292-653

$17.95

DEDICATION

To everyone who has type 2 diabetes.
Follow the cloud of God's presence and
know He will show you the way.

PROLOGUE

Christy Fielding felt light-headed as Chuck walked her across the compound to the infirmary. She held onto his arm for balance, but she was breathing hard when they arrived. She never tried to delay their arrival and cooperated because she didn't believe she had any other choice. She didn't know that night she was walking to her death. Unlike someone sentenced to death by the courts, her protest would not have mattered. She was a prisoner who had been held captive for months.

When they arrived at the infirmary, Chuck helped her onto a table and returned with supplies to start an intravenous line in her forearm. She couldn't lie down until he brought two pillows to hold her more upright. The symptom told Chuck his patient was in heart failure from anemia.

"You're the only good part of this, Chuck," she said as he rolled a tank of nitrous oxide to her bedside. "You don't have to be kind to me, but you always are."

Chuck looked at her, trying not to remember she was only twenty. He was sure the constant blood donations he had been taking from her were killing her. Christy was very fair skinned like anyone with red hair, but her skin was white from anemia. When he looked at her face, he felt like her eyes could see inside his soul.

"I forgive you, Chuck," she said gently. "I know this isn't your fault. You have to do it. God will forgive you if you just ask him. I pray for you every day."

He pressed the mask to her face to stop her words. He couldn't stand hearing her acceptance of her impending death when he would be her executioner. She had no idea he had killed dozens of people before her.

"Breathe deep, Christy, and go to sleep. I have to get started."

She wasn't afraid because she didn't know it was to be the last time she would ever go to sleep. He put the needle in her limp arm and drew a sample to test her red blood count. It was only 18%. Normal for her age would have been 38%. She had been bled almost to death by him. As he looked at the reading, all the deaths he had caused overwhelmed Chuck.

"How long will it take, Chuck?" his supervisor asked from the door.

"Two or three hours if you really want it all."

"Every drop," the supervisor replied. "The old man has a surgery scheduled for this week."

Chuck nodded and bent over Christy as if he was going to obey orders, but the supervisor had pushed Chuck to make a decision he had considered for weeks. He had decided he would let Christy live no matter what the price. He could not know he was the instrument to answer her fervent prayers for rescue.

When his supervisor had disappeared down the corridor, Chuck prepared the bed next to Christy's as if he had another patient coming. He took the corpse that was awaiting transport in the refrigeration unit to lie in that bed. He taped an IV to the body and covered it. Then he wrapped the head in a towel and transferred the gas mask to the dead face. Within minutes of the gas mask's removal, Christy began to awaken. Chuck pulled the needle from her arm roughly to speed the process.

"Wake up, Christy. We've got to get out of here." She looked at him with sleep bemused eyes.

"Chuck, are you finished?"

He tied a dressing around her arm tightly and dimmed the lights in the room. "Get up, Christy. We've got to get out of here. I need you to be really quiet and hurry. He dumped the linens into the dirty utility room and inverted the laundry bag. "Get in this bag so I can hide you."

"Why?" She was still too sedated to comprehend what was happening. She sat up slowly and saw the body in the bed beside her. There was no mistaking that it was a corpse. It was a girl Christy had known for two years.

"Bernice?" she gasped. "Chuck, is it Bernice?"

"She's dead, Christy. She was killed for her blood. You will be, too, and so will I if you don't do everything I say. Get in the bag and don't make a sound."

Christy had never been so frightened, but she obeyed Chuck because she had prayed Chuck would rescue her. She had trusted him even though he had helped hold her hostage and had helped to bleed her almost to death. She was praying as she laid limply across Chuck's shoulder. The feel of his footsteps told her when they were out of the compound and crossing the parking lot. He stopped at the far edge of the gravel lot to release her. As he pulled the bag away, sirens alarmed, and every light in the compound came on.

"They know! They know what I've done," Chuck said hysterically. "Run for my car. It's the black convertible."

Christy ran as fast as she could, but she was in heart failure because of her anemia. She ran out of breath before she had crossed half the distance. She stumbled, and Chuck picked her up and carried her the rest of the way. Her pulse was roaring in her ears, but she could hear a loud popping around them. Just as they reached the car, she felt Chuck jerk and fall down. He threw her the keys.

"Get away, Christy. They're coming."

"Not without you," she said. She unlocked the car with fumbling hands and opened it with difficulty. Then, she half dragged Chuck to his feet and shoved him into the passenger side. It was too dark for her to see the blood and know he had been shot.

She slammed the door and got into the driver's seat, starting the car before she closed the door. She floored the gas pedal and drove out of the parking lot, spraying gravel in their wake.

"Put on your seat belt, Chuck," she ordered him. "Which way is out?"

"That road. When it dead ends, turn right." He looked at Christy knowing he was badly wounded and still could not regret his decision. He knew sparing her life was worth his own. He only hoped that sacrifice would buy him forgiveness from all the other deaths.

"Where's your house, Chuck?" she asked. "We can go there and call the police."

"It's about twenty miles from here, Christy, but they may already be there." He tried to look back and the pain in his back worsened to the point that he couldn't bear it.

They reached the main highway as Chuck groaned in pain, and Christy remained on the dirt road as she reached out to him.

"Drive," he demanded. "Drive or they'll catch us. They have too much at stake to let us live."

"What is at stake?" she begged as she sped down the state highway. The moon was shining in her window as if to light her way, but she stared at the road ahead of them and at Chuck. "Why are they doing this?"

"The Divilbiss family is incredibly rich. They're millionaires. They have a clotting problem kind of like hemophilia. When people started catching AIDS and hepatitis from blood products, they decided to grow their own. They have AB- blood so they look for people with that blood type, using the blood drives to find them. They harvest blood until your bodies can't take the stress anymore, and then we take all the blood out until you die. God forgive me. I've been taking the blood. Tonight I was supposed to kill you. I couldn't do it."

He made an effort to breathe as the pain in his back wound tighter. "My house is fifteen miles down this road, but you need to pull off just beyond it so we can make sure it's safe. You may not be able to get help from the police, Christy. Rich people can buy anything they want.

They can buy people. If anyone is at my house, get back on the state highway and drive toward the interstate. Keep driving, and when you leave the car, change your name and hide. If your name is in a computer anywhere, they might find you."

He was silent until the side road appeared ahead of them, and then he pointed to it. "Cut the lights and turn there."

They pulled onto the dark side street and looked down at the quiet street. There were four cars in the driveway facing them, and Chuck shook his head. "They're already there. Head for the interstate. Don't break any traffic laws but drive as fast as you can." He fumbled to reach into his jacket pocket and retrieved a driver's license and a folded paper as well as the snack money he carried. "That's your ID. They were going to destroy it. Your family thinks you're dead already." He drew a deep, shuddering breath and said, "God forgive me. Please, God, forgive me."

Christy was completely terrified then, and she drove with her whole being focused on the road, the speedometer, and the rear view mirror. She knew Chuck was hurt and couldn't help her anymore. She didn't have anyone else to help her either. She had been chosen by the Divilbiss family for just that reason.

She looked up once and saw a brightly painted water tower that looked like a Halloween jack-o-lantern. She felt as if even that false face was jeering at her. She reached the interstate at 9:30 P.M. and saw the sign pointing west to Oak Ridge. The other sign directed her east to Knoxville. She turned east and drove at seventy miles an hour until the rest stop just before Knoxville. She pulled into a parking place and touched Chuck. That one touch told her he was dead.

Christy had never felt as alone as she felt that night sitting in the rest area with a dead man. She tried to pray, but the terror was too great. Finally, she rested her head on the steering wheel and cried until every emotion within her had been spent. It was morning before she could make herself get out of the car. She wiped the steering wheel and covered Chuck with the blanket from the back seat. Then she threw the car keys in the floorboard and ran over to where the trucks were parked. "I'm broke down," she said to the nearest trucker. "Can you give me a ride into Knoxville?"

"Sure, kid. Hop in," said the trucker. "You aren't a runaway, are you?"

"Not me," Christy lied. "I'm on my way home." She did not add that she didn't know where home would be.

CHAPTER 1

Gabe Killian had good endurance, but he was drenched in sweat when he and his class reached the convenience store at Deep Creek Campground. He had hiked his environmental biology students twenty-seven miles that day, and he wished he could hike them back up the hill and into the creek to cool off. His students stormed the building to buy sodas, bottled water, and various snacks. Normally, Gabe would have followed them into the store and lectured them on the harmful effects of excess sugar and fat intake and its contribution to the epidemic of diabetes in America. The students were spared the lecture because their teacher was also seeking a drink. He didn't really want to go in the store and see the things that would always tempt him. He had made a commitment to a healthy lifestyle and hoped living that commitment would protect him from diabetes. He also hoped his public statements might persuade some of his acquaintances and students to do the same.

Gabe went to the outside water faucet and threw water on his face and neck before refilling his canteen and pouring it down his back. He drank from the second refill and was refilling his canteen a third time when he heard footsteps behind him.

"You need more sunscreen," a female voice observed.

Gabe turned to see a pretty but sober-faced girl watching him. She had obviously been stacking inner tubes. He surmised she worked for the camping part of the convenience store.

"I don't usually burn," he said dubiously. "Where is it?"

"The back of your neck." She pulled a tube of sunscreen from her shorts pocket. "Use this. It's 50 spf." He smiled at her as he took the tube, noticing she had bright auburn hair and the very fair skin to go with it. Her complexion explained why she was carrying the tube. Her face seemed to hold his gaze like a magnet. He found himself powerless to look away. Gabe applied the sunscreen to his neck while struggling to make conversation. He was rarely at a loss for words.

"This is proof the sun can get to anyone's skin," he said as he recapped the tube. "I guess I haven't been in the full sun enough to get a base tan on my back yet. By the end of the summer you won't need to ask if I live on the reservation." He extended the tube slowly. "Thanks. I don't want to be the first Cherokee to have skin cancer."

The girl took the tube and tucked it into her pocket. It bothered Gabe that she was still unsmiling. He had expected his joke might ease the natural tension between two strangers. But his only reward was her continued interest.

"Are you a tour guide?" she asked.

"I teach at the college outside of Cherokee," Gabe said. "This is the lab for my environmental biology class. We'll be through here several times before August." He extended his hand to the girl. "I'm Gabe Killian. Do you work here? I don't remember seeing you, and I come through here periodically when I'm not teaching." She shook his hand tentatively and was rewarded by a sudden feeling of magnetic connection. It was so strong that she kept his fingers for a long moment. She was blushing when she released his hand. Gabe was likewise mesmerized by the sensation and didn't notice her embarrassment.

"I'm Christy," she said. "I do tube rentals so I don't do much business with hikers."

Gabe wasn't usually attracted to white women, but touching Christy had engendered a feeling he had never experienced. He had a vivid impression that he had been destined to meet her. He pushed ahead in an effort to get to know her

"You never know," he said. "Environmental biology does cover the water. Tubing might be a good way to observe underwater life forms."

"Later in the summer you might," she said seriously. "When the current slows down, you can just float downstream until you get to the waterfalls. Right now it's a pretty fast ride." She turned back to the tubes abruptly as her boss glanced out of the store window. Gabe felt curiously shunned and walked away. His students were trickling out of the store, and he felt uncomfortable talking to Christy in their presence. He and his class took seats in the shade to wait for their bus back to the campus.

After a few minutes, he couldn't keep from watching the pretty redhead. He guessed she was around twenty years old, and standing near her had told him she was no more than five feet three inches in height. She was small boned and slender, but she lifted the heavy inner tubes with the ease of trained muscles. At the same time, she was too thin to be healthy. She was also very pale. She was wearing a worn denim shirt tied like a halter with the sleeves cut out and a pair of blue jean cut off shorts. Her hair was braided and fell to her waist. She had crystalline blue eyes and a smattering of freckles on her nose and shoulders. She wasn't wearing any jewelry.

"And what sort of life form are you assessing now, Dr. Killian?" Josh Turney teased him.

"I'm just planning the next hike, Josh." Gabe shrugged. "Maybe we'll finish off our next twenty-seven miles with a nice tube ride."

"I think the professor has a conflict of interest," Josh announced to the rest of the class. Gabe ignored the banter partially because he didn't feel comfortable with his own response to the girl. Most of the class, especially the female students, also ignored it for different reasons.

The bus ride back to Cherokee took thirty minutes, and Gabe took the opportunity to give his class their homework while they were held captive. When the bus doors opened, his class dispersed quickly. Gabe shouldered his pack and hiked across campus to his pickup truck. He found his cousin and roommate, Job, lying in the truck bed. Gabe discovered this when he threw his backpack on top of Job.

"What the heck are you doing?" Job exclaimed as he sat up. "You almost killed me, man."

Gabe opened the passenger door and walked around to the driver's side. "I'm here to remind you that you ought to be studying instead of sleeping, Job."

"I worked until midnight, Gabe. Give me a break. Even computers get to sleep occasionally." He vaulted over the side and slid into the passenger's seat. "You need a shower."

"Really? I hadn't noticed." Gabe started the engine and rolled down his window. "Did you check the fridge this morning?"

"The cupboard's bare, man. Drop me at the corner market, and give me a twenty. I'll get us some supper." Gabe dug into his wallet at the next traffic light and passed two twenty dollar bills to Job.

"No junk food, please. There are plenty of diabetic Cherokee already. Let's not make two more." Job rolled his eyes and stuffed the money into his jeans.

"You're obsessed with this diabetes thing, Gabe. My theory is you're just jealous because you're getting too old to burn the good stuff off."

"Keep it up, cousin, and you'll be burning it off by walking home every day. You're just gloating because your side of the family doesn't have diabetes yet. You're still at risk, and we both know it. This is one of the sugar capitals of the known world." Gabe pulled into the parking lot of a small grocery and let Job out at the door. Five minutes later he pulled into their driveway.

Gabe's house was his inheritance from his mother, Raynelle. She had died three years earlier from a heart attack. Her heart condition had resulted from uncontrolled type 2 diabetes. Watching his mother die had made Gabe very concerned about his own risk for the disease. It was rampant in Native American people and spreading like a plague across America. He knew he would probably develop diabetes eventually, but Gabe was determined not to hurry the process by eating unhealthy foods and gaining weight. He had also started preaching the dangers of eating sugar and fat and the lack of exercise to everyone he knew.

He was an only child and had never known his father. Seaman Adam Killian had died in Vietnam when his son had been eight months old. The house had seemed very empty to Gabe when his mother's funeral was over. He had invited Job to live with him as insulation against loneliness. Job had filled a huge void in his life since then.

The house was a neat brick rectangle with a screen porch in back and vine covered trellises surrounding the front porch. Gabe sat in the shade of the trellises to flip through his mail before heading for the shower. Standing under the water, he thought of Christy and his life history of superficial relationships. He had never let a girl get close to him emotionally, but he had also never wanted to take the risk. When he thought of Christy, it seemed essential to get to know her better. He told himself she had given him ample reason to believe she was unattainable. Even the prospect of being brushed off couldn't keep his thoughts off her. He found it impossible to analyze why seeing her seemed so important. He thought it was because their eyes had been locked together for so many minutes. He told himself it might just be the scent hormones biologists talked about. As he toweled himself and dressed, he decided to *act* and not analyze his feelings. It was a first for him.

Gabe was scrubbed, dressed and had started a load of laundry when Job kicked the front door to ask for admittance. That mode of arrival always annoyed Gabe who had obsessive-compulsive disorder about his house. It was always clean, and even nicks in the varnished front door could send him to the hardware store.

"Can't you learn to knock like a human, Job?" His twenty-year-old cousin grinned endearingly.

"Full arms, man. I'm pleased to report I have all sorts of nutritious, nonfattening stuff, no sugar, and no alcohol. You'll have to weigh that against the door."

Gabe stood back to admit Job and then took one of the two sacks and followed him to the kitchen to unload. Job had not lied. The sacks were full of fresh produce, bread, skim milk, and a package of hamburger.

"Okay, you have chosen wisely. I'll let you off on the door just this once. You know I'm lecturing you for your own good."

"I know," Job said. "And I know why. I'm just giving you a hard time. Hey, I stopped drinking soda just for you."

Gabe grinned and patted Job on the back. He started unloading the groceries and then thought of Christy again. "Does it look like the back of my neck got sun-burned, Job?"

"You're kidding, right?" Job examined Gabe's neck. "You don't have any hope of becoming a redneck as far as I can tell. Why?" Gabe grinned. Job's response gave him the impression Christy had been flirting with him.

"No particular reason. I just wondered."

"Eat something. I think your blood sugar must be low," Job said.

Chapter 2

Gabe and Job had supper and talked about Job's classes and Gabe's hike through Deep Creek. Job finished the evening by taking his books to his girlfriend's house while Gabe sat down with his classroom planner and stared off into space. He was thirty-one, and he felt as if he had reached some sort of critical point in his life. Following in his father's footsteps, he had left the reservation at seventeen to join the Navy. His commanding officers had made most of his decisions until he had graduated and become an officer. Early in his career, he had chosen to become a member of the Seal teams, the elite Navy special forces. It had not been an easy goal, but as a Seal, he had felt invincible and in control of his life. The other men on his team had been his family. He had expected the Navy would be his life's work.

His destiny was obviously down another road. He had been twenty-six when a mission had left him with a depressed skull fracture. The doctors said he should have died and to be thankful that he had only lost some vision.

"You'll have to transfer, Lieutenant Killian," his commanding officer had told him. "Navy Seals can't afford any loss of peripheral vision. How could you defend yourself and the other team members?"

Gabe had known without asking that he would be assigned to an administrative post. Being trapped at a desk just wasn't an option for him. He had taken a medical discharge and used his access to the GI bill. Since he had graduated from college while in the Navy, he had applied and been accepted to graduate school. He had completed his Ph.D. in three years and started teaching. Dr. Gabriel Killian was progressing very well in his career, but his career was the scope of his life. Some part of him wanted more, especially at night when he was alone with his thoughts.

Remembering things he still regretted left Gabe unable to concentrate. Finally he gave up on his lesson plans and left the house at eight o'clock. He jogged to the church where Job's father was the preacher. He had decided not to use his car for any distance less than a mile because he knew exercise was key in reducing his body's use of insulin. Resistance to insulin was what he had inherited that put him at risk for diabetes. He understood that insulin resistance meant his body had to make much more insulin to use the foods he ate as fuel. He also understood that using too much insulin would eventually cause his pancreas to run out of insulin. Exercise let his body use food without needing insulin. He tried to run every night after supper to burn off that meal. The run to see Jonah Killian had a dual purpose.

As usual, Jonah Killian was running a study hall for Cherokee children whose parents worked nights. His uncle grinned broadly on seeing him.

"Gabe, how are you?" He studied his nephew's face and saw Gabe was troubled.

"Can I bend your ear, Jonah?" Jonah nodded sagely and led Gabe to his makeshift desk in the corner.

"You haven't bent my ear in some time now, but I've been expecting you." There was a long silence while Gabe thought of Christy and how to begin the discussion.

"I met a girl I'd like to get to know better."

"It's time," Jonah said. "You should have your own family."

"She's white," Gabe said. He was relieved when Jonah's face never changed.

"I'm not so given to tribal purity as others. I've always believed God chooses the right person for everyone. You aren't making a decision about the rest of your life by dating her."

"You always make everything sound easy," Gabe said. "It's easy to think you know what God wants. It's hard to be sure."

"If you don't take the chance of looking, Gabe, you'll never see what He has planned for you." He scanned his nephew's face. "Your mother's mistake isn't your legacy."

"You're the only man who can say that to me and not sound like a psychologist." Gabe sat back and looked at the room full of children. He enjoyed working with children, but he hadn't ever let himself believe he could have his own. He had issues that clouded his ability to look for a wife, but he never tried to get past them because he felt they couldn't be resolved. Jonah put his hand on Gabe's arm and interrupted the negative thoughts.

"Someday, we need to talk about the past and not just the future. When I see you coming through the door, I always hope it will be the day. There are feelings you need to put behind you."

"I don't dwell on what I can't change, Jonah. That isn't healthy." He paused. "She's about twenty years old. Do you think that's too young? I kind of feel like I'm asking one of my students out."

"Stop looking for reasons not to see her, Gabe," Jonah chided. "You find her attractive. It's natural to want to know her better. When you do, you'll learn if your relationship is meant to be more. Only one woman affected me this way. She touched my heart from the first moment I went out with her. Ultimately, I made her my wife."

"It was very different meeting Christy," Gabe admitted. "I had this strange feeling that I already knew her. Right now, I'm obsessed with seeing her again. I don't know whether to be pleased or frightened."

"Finding your soul mate is a gift, Gabe. It isn't impossible that she's the one God made for you." He scanned Gabe's face. "My father was eleven years older than my mother. When they met he was thirty years old, and she was nineteen. He was a cautious man and not quick to bare his soul or open his heart. My father's name was Gabriel. I believe you knew him."

"Yeah," Gabe smiled. "I remember him. I'd like to think someday I might earn the honor of having his name. Thanks for listening, Jonah. I guess I'll be driving up to Deep Creek tomorrow. I'll let you know how it turns out."

As he left, he passed the sons and daughters of men his age and thought of the family he wanted and didn't have. He was a part of Jonah's family, but he had always wanted that kind of relationship with his own wife and children. He felt as if the unknown girl were his last and only chance to have his dream.

Running at dusk in Cherokee was safe even in 1999. Gabe had black belts in three forms of martial arts. His body told the people who didn't know. He was six feet tall and had little visible body fat even though he was stockier and fifteen pounds heavier than he had been in the service. His upper body advertised that he could bench press two hundred fifty pounds. He had met more than a few unattached women while running, but Christy NoLastName kept his memory's attention while he ran that night. He thought of her until he went to sleep and awakened with clear intentions.

Fridays in the summer were days Gabe worked for the National Park Service as a field botanist. He chose to spend Friday, June 11 at Deep Creek Campground. He started the day at the convenience store under the guise of buying bottled water, but Christy wasn't there. Deep Creek was outside of Cherokee so Gabe didn't know the owner. He couldn't ask where Christy was without drawing attention to himself. Nonetheless, his appearance drew the attention of the other female employees. They watched him walking down the trail until he disappeared from view.

Christy was scrubbing the camper shower stalls and toilets. It was the least favorite task of the girls working the campground. They drew lots for who had to do it. Christy lost frequently, but she didn't complain. When she returned to the rental equipment, no one mentioned that Gabe had come because they didn't know his name. They often talked about attractive men passing through their area. She didn't know the man she had thought about all night was the subject of that day's discussion. When the others were grading the guys that day, she daydreamed about Gabe.

Gabe spent the morning in the forest cataloging pitcher plants, an endangered species. He emerged at two o'clock for a belated lunch and the chance to see Christy. She was at the tube station as he reached the store. He hesitated when he saw the unforgettable auburn braid. Christy felt the same hesitation when she saw him, but she raised her hand somberly. Gabe grinned and raised his hand in a time honored movie gesture.

"How!" He was pleased when Christy smiled. "You know I've always wondered why they chose *how* instead of who or what."

"Didn't you lose your sheep?" she asked just suppressing a laugh.

"That's a once a week class," Gabe said. "I get eight hours to demoralize them every Wednesday. They have to rest up for a week afterwards." He put down his pack and emptied the hot dregs from his canteen. He was reassured when she continued to lean against the inner tubes watching him.

"So, what was today? Homework?"

Gabe turned on the outside faucet and refilled his canteen. "I have two jobs. I teach, and I do field biology work for the National Park Service. Today I'm surveying carnivorous plants." Her smile was tremulous as if she had not smiled in months.

"Aren't you afraid? You might be eaten on the job."

"You're thinking Little Shop of Horrors," Gabe said. "If you can take a break, I'll show you what I'm talking about." There was a long pause when Gabe mentally willed Christy to agree. She finally nodded almost reluctantly.

"I only get fifteen minutes so this had better be close." She made her excuses to the owner and then followed Gabe off the hiking trail and up into a thick deciduous forest. They sidestepped down to a small tributary of Deep Creek, and Gabe knelt in the swampy grass to indicate a small tubular plant.

"This is a pitcher plant. It's also known as Sarracenia. This particular one is called Dixie Lace. It's an endangered species because unscrupulous gardeners and nurseries dig them up even in protected areas to propagate them and sell them. The government considers plant poaching to be a bad thing so they hire field biologists to keep an estimate of the density in the national parks."

"Sometimes I think humans are born to destroy things." Christy knelt down close to him and touched the fringed mouth of the tube delicately. Everything about her seemed as rare and special as the endangered plant. She glanced at Gabe. "It's so fragile. What does it eat?"

"Small insects. It's similar to the Venus fly trap." He brushed the mouth with his fingertip. The plant seemed to move in response. More than the movement, the gentleness of Gabe Killian's hands was surprising to Christy. She thought men who could be gentle were also endangered.

"It's going to be very disappointed when it realizes it hasn't caught its dinner," Gabe said.

"Are you a specialist in this kind of stuff?" Christy asked.

"I have my doctorate in biology. It's the perfect job. I'm paid to go hiking. I don't do well with confinement. My least favorite days are the dress clothes, tie, behind my desk days."

"This part could be a drag in January," she observed. "It's really cold up here in the winter."

"That's when you light a fire in the fireplace and indulge in hot tea after walking in the snow." He looked into her eyes and was pleased when she didn't look away. "Some people use shared body warmth to stay comfortable during the cold weather." It was a subtle advance. He intended it to see if she was interested in getting to know him. Christy didn't know how to respond even though she had wanted to meet Gabe the first time she saw him.

"Well, it's a long time until winter," she said. "Have you got the time?" Gabe hid his face from her as they stood because he felt certain that Christy was telling him to back off. The rejection affected him more than he thought it should have.

"You've got about five more minutes." He started down the mountainside moving briskly. It was a moment when Christy had to make a choice of trusting Gabe Killian or losing the chance of knowing him. She reached out for the first time since her desperate flight for survival. Gabe was startled when she touched his arm like the brush of a butterfly's wings.

"Are you carnivorous too? I guess I should have asked before I went walking with you." Her words were a clear invitation to continue their interaction.

"Yeah. Actually I am, but I'd have to cook you first. I don't eat anything warm blooded in its raw state." He saw she was smiling and took that encouragement to press ahead. "If you go out to supper with me, we'd both be properly fed and then you wouldn't be at any risk until the next meal time." She hesitated for twenty yards while Gabe wondered if she might have a problem dating a Cherokee. Her reply surprised him.

"I don't have any dress-up clothes anymore. I lost all my things last year just before I came here. All I have are clothes like this."

"Like I said, I'm not a dress-up kind of guy. There's a restaurant over in Cherokee with a balcony over the river. Shorts and tee shirts don't bother them. Let's go eat there. I'll be working until six."

"So will I," Christy said slowly. "I'll wait for you, but just so you know, I live back in the woods so I can't stay out too late. It's too hard to get up the road at night."

"I promise, Cinderella. You'll be home way before midnight."

They parted company at the dirt road, and Gabe hiked deeper into woods elated with success.

Christy returned to the inner tubes soberly but feeling something akin to happiness. It seemed a very alien sensation because she had not felt it for so very long. Her coworker, Joannie Parker, sidled up beside her.

"Who's the guy, Christy?"

"His name is Gabe Killian. He's a teacher from the college over in Cherokee," Christy said. "He asked me out."

"If you decide not to go, let me know," Joannie offered. "I could be tempted by the body or the face." She scanned Christy's face. "You aren't really even interested, are you? That guy is totally hot."

"I'm interested. I just don't know if I want to be involved with anybody. I got my heart broken last year, and I'm not really over it. And I don't really know anything about him. It's risky to go out with a stranger."

"Ask Bo about him. He knows everybody in North Carolina," Joannie suggested. "If you don't, I will because he might look my way if you don't look his way."

Christy walked away to avoid further questions, but she couldn't stop thinking about Gabe so easily. Joannie's threat to pursue him made Christy nervous because she was interested. Gabe Killian was attractive in a different way than any man she had known. She had correctly guessed he was about thirty. She was impressed because he was in excellent physical shape. His copper complexion had told her he was Cherokee before he had. He had thick, jet black hair that rose in a widow's peak on the left side of his forehead and fell to the nape of his neck. His eyes were such a dark brown that they looked black. Christy had never met a man with such beautiful eyes.

Christy hadn't intended to accept anyone's offer because she had too many secrets to keep. Still, she had very spontaneously made an overture to the handsome Cherokee teacher. Gabe had made it impossible to refuse his offer for supper because she sensed in him a kindred spirit. She knew intuitively that he was a man who had his own secrets perhaps as painful as her own. Her only concern was how to go on a date when he might find out where she was living and other things she could not explain.

CHAPTER 3

Gabe showed up at six o'clock on the dot. The convenience store was closing for the night, and the crowds around it had thinned. Joannie saw Gabe first and came to quiz Christy.

"Did you decide, Christy? I'm totally ready to make a pass at him if you aren't," Joannie whispered.

"What did Bo say?" Christy asked nervously. She hadn't been able to keep her mind off Gabe Killian, but she was still unnerved by the prospects of a date.

"According to Bo's sources, everyone in Cherokee knows him. He's supposed to be a super nice guy." Joannie unbuttoned the top two buttons of her halter top, displaying her enviable anatomy. She removed her ponytail band and shook out her long dark hair.

"He asked me out," Christy said defiantly. "I want to go out with him. When he decides I'm not worth the time, you can come on to him."

"Maybe I ought to stay around," Joannie said. "With that kind of attitude, you won't be a fun date." She glanced back at the road and waved at Gabe before returning to her tubes. Christy attacked her own pile of just returned inner tubes in an effort to hide her nervousness. She shuddered when she saw her reflection in a puddle as she heard him behind her. Her face and shoulders were smeared with mud. When she turned to meet Gabe, she had the expression of a little girl caught in mischief.

"I'm sorry. I just realized I'm a mess." She expected his gaze to make her feel worse, but Gabe just smiled and shrugged.

"You can't be much dirtier than I am. It just shows up more on your skin. Let's go up to the waterfall, and we can both wash off. We'll be dry by the time we get to Cherokee."

"What about your car?" she asked.

"In my line of work, it pays to have seat covers." He left her to put his pack into a burgundy truck and took out two towels before relocking it. "I'm ready when you are, Christine."

"It's Christianna. My mother was Swedish." She brushed her hands on her shorts. "I always say that with trepidation because most guys immediately assume Swedish girls are easy and cheap. I'm not either."

"If I thought you were, I wouldn't be asking you out. A guy my age isn't just looking for a good time. You look like the kind of girl who has always looked for more than that." She looked enchanting as he gave her one of the towels. "I'll race you to the showers."

She surprised him with how fast she could run up the grade to Tom Branch falls. She kept pace with him until they were splashing into the place where Deep Creek widened into a pool. It was only three feet at its deepest point, and the water was pleasantly cool to people who had worked all day in June's humidity. Climbing up on the waterfall's base allowed them to stand beneath nature's shower.

"You must be a runner," Gabe said. He tossed his towel onto a rock.

"I ran track in high school," she said breathlessly. "I wasn't fast enough for a track scholarship, but I love to run." She put her towel beside his and stood under the waterfall. He wasn't breathless at all, but Christy knew her body hadn't recovered from the chronic blood loss. She couldn't afford vitamins. She could barely afford food.

"How did you get so fast?" she asked.

"The Navy. For a water-based military force, they love to see you run on dry land. Of course, they also like to see you run in sand and on the beach and in the water. If they had paid me in mileage, I'd be seriously rich now." He turned his face into the water and scrubbed his hair. Then he pulled off his tank top to rinse it in the pool. Christy's eyes were drawn to his body because it was so attractive. That was not what had originally caught her eye, but he was a handsome man. His dark skin rippled over his muscles as he washed the grime off his chest and back.

"How long were you in the Navy?" she asked.

"Nine years. The Navy was my career until I was injured. Then I used my GI bill to go to graduate school and become a professional hiker." She stared at him more openly as she wondered what his job had been. He answered as if he could hear her thoughts.

"I was a Seal. That's a member of the Navy's special forces teams. I hope that doesn't lower your belief in our country's defense system too much."

"I'm impressed," she said genuinely. "I feel incredibly safe. I'll bet you know every form of martial arts on the planet."

"I concentrate on taekwondo, kung fu and jujitsu. Martial arts are more than a method of defense. They keep you focused. Kind of a 'use the force' form of concentration. I'd be willing to give you some free lessons."

"I'd like to learn," she admitted. "You never know when you might get hassled. I don't have any way to protect myself." She turned her back on him pretending she had turned to scrub the front of her tee shirt. Her fear had returned in a sudden rush, and she didn't want him to see it.

"I've only been here since last fall. I got involved in an abusive relationship, and I had to leave."

"I've been in one of those," Gabe admitted. "Sometimes all the martial arts on the planet can't protect you from being abused." He put his hand on her shoulder. Her skin was strikingly soft. Touching her gave him a rush of protectiveness. "I'd be happy to protect you from the physical kind."

She put her hand over his hand without turning. "I'd like to feel safe, Gabe. I haven't felt safe in a long time."

Gabe put his other hand on her opposite shoulder and pulled her back against his body in a very spontaneous embrace. He was startled by what he had done but forgot to think about it when she relaxed against him. It felt very natural to hold her in the soft darkness of early evening. Her body seemed to fit perfectly in his arms.

Christy closed her eyes and reveled in the moment of feeling safe and no longer alone in an unfriendly world. Reality returned abruptly as a group of teenagers ran past the waterfall. She stepped away from Gabe.

"I guess I'm as clean as I can get," she said. Gabe offered her his hand as they clambered through the current toward the bank. Christy tentatively extended her hand to meet his. When his hand closed around hers, she felt another magnetic current between them urging her to move closer. She had never felt such a powerful attraction to a man. They walked back to the truck holding hands and listening to the coming of night.

It was still very warm as they drove back to Cherokee, but even with the windows down, their clothes were damp when they reached the outskirts of town.

"Well, we may need to rethink the timing of supper," Gabe admitted. "Let me loan you a tee shirt and a pair of shorts. I live a half mile from the restaurant, and my cousin, Job, will be at the house so you don't have to worry about ulterior motives."

She nodded acceptance and continued surveying the town. "I don't have a car so I haven't seen Cherokee until today. Were you born here?"

"I was born on the naval base in Virginia Beach. My father was drafted to Vietnam so he enlisted in the Navy. Most of the men in our family have served in the Navy since World War II. My father was the equivalent of a Seal. They used to call it the underwater demolition team. He was killed when I was eight months old. Actually, he was missing in action for about six months so my mother stayed on the base at Virginia Beach. By the time they declared my father dead, she had gotten involved with another man. She married him, and we lived on the base until I was six. We moved here after my stepfather died. All of my parents' relatives are here. My father's brother is a preacher, and he was my surrogate father."

"Does your mother still live here?"

"She died three years ago. She was diabetic, and she had all the bad complications. She died from a heart attack." Gabe's face told Christy that his mother's death was still just a little too close for comfort. "I was her only child so it was hard. I asked Job to move in because it was too quiet." He smiled to dispel the somber air. "It hasn't been quiet since he came. Job is quite a character. You'll like him."

"If he's like you, I'm sure I will," she said.

"Where's your family?" He felt a deeper kinship with her when he saw Christy was keeping her eyes forcefully on the scenery.

"My parents were killed in a car accident when I was three. My father was a missionary. He met my mother while he was working with a church in Africa. She was an aid worker from Sweden. He had to learn Swedish to talk to her. I was born in the Congo. There was a long period of bad political instability, and the missionaries had to leave. We were in Germany when my parents were killed. My dad's mother brought me to Tennessee and raised me until she died when I was fifteen. The people in our church took care of me after that, but I was sort of passed around from family to family. I always felt like I was somebody's Christian duty so I left when I was eighteen." She shrugged. "I guess we can have a competition for the saddest tale, but I fully expect to win."

"Hey, I thought my story was pretty darn depressing." He pulled into his driveway and switched off the ignition. "Here we are. The Castle Killian."

"It's really nice," she said wistfully. "It reminds me of my grandma's house."

"It was my grandmother's house," Gabe told her. He opened the truck door for her and then took her hand to escort her to the house. He unlocked the house and stepped in, calling for Job. When there was no answer, he said, "I guess he's out with Darla, his girlfriend. If you'd rather, you can wait on the porch until I change."

Christy closed the door without any reservations. It had the quietly comfortable look afforded by polished 1940 era furniture. Everything about Gabe's house made her feel strangely at home. "I trust you. I'll just wait here."

"I won't be long. Make yourself comfortable. There's iced tea and milk in the fridge." He left nonchalantly but hustled when he was out of sight. Getting ready involved a very fast shower and a clean tank top and jeans. He searched through his clothes to find a new tee shirt and the smallest pair of shorts he owned for Christy. When he returned to the living room, he found her examining his books and tapes.

"I wouldn't have figured you for a Windham Hill fan," she said. "I used to listen to George Winston for hours at a time. Can I put one on?"

"Make yourself at home," he said. He was struck by how much they had in common. She seemed to fit so perfectly into his life. Impulsively, Gabe bent to kiss her.

The kiss was unexpected for Christy. For a brief instant, she stiffened until the magnetic attraction between them overpowered every other thought in her mind. Then, she melted into the feelings he had engendered. They moved closer together until their bodies were touching. Gabe continued holding her as the kiss ended. He was startled by how quickly he had felt desire for even more physical contact. He was pleased when she didn't move away.

"I almost forgot about supper for a minute," he said.

"I guess I'd better get changed." She held onto his arm almost as if she were incapable of letting go. It was hard to think of what to say when her heart was fluttering in her chest. "Did you find some clothes I can wear?"

"I found a shirt that may be big enough to be a dress. I left everything on the bathroom counter. I'll put on George Winston while you're dressing. If you want to take a real shower, I left out a clean towel."

She did want a shower, and she wanted to look good for Gabe Killian. She scrubbed her hair and body with the soap and shampoo she found in the shower. She found a hair dryer in the bathroom closet and used it to dry her hair. It was impossible to look feminine in the tee shirt and shorts, but she hoped he would overlook the clothes. She was leaving the bathroom when she decided it might be better if she tried to impress him in other ways.

Gabe had flipped through his George Winston collection until he found the CD, "Forest." He sat down to listen with a glass of ice water beside him. When he closed his eyes, Christy's face immediately came into his mind, and he allowed himself to think what it would be like to marry her. Instead of being relaxed by the image and the music, he had a flashback to the day his stepfather had died. Christy's hand on his shoulder startled him out of his thoughts. He came to his feet abruptly, hoping she wouldn't notice the remembered fear and rage on his face.

"Sometimes I do that, too," Christy said slowly. "Sometimes when bad things happen to you, they get a life of their own. That's why I haven't gone out in a long time. It's always there keeping me alone."

Gabe looked at her with fascination. He had been sent to therapy for years and had never felt anyone had empathy with him.

"You do understand," he said in surprise.

"I do understand," Christy confirmed. "I used to be afraid to go to sleep because then I knew I would dream." She hesitated. "I just want to think happy thoughts tonight. I was thinking I could cook supper for you. After all, I don't look as nice as I would like to look when we do go out. I'm just wondering if you have food in your fridge. Sometimes bachelors don't keep much besides beer and cookies."

"I don't drink alcohol, and I try not to eat sugar or junk food because there's so much diabetes in my family," he replied. "I also like to cook so I actually try to keep food here. Since Job eats more than the average black bear, I'm not always successful." He looked into the refrigerator and nodded with relief. "We have eggs, cheese, milk, and vegetables."

She made two vegetable omelets and a big salad. Gabe made a pot of hot tea and then sat watching her with great appreciation as she prepared their supper. No one other than Reba and his mother had ever cooked for him. It made him feel as if he had really come home that night.

"I don't know your last name," he said.

"It's Fielding. I didn't know if I wanted to tell you," Christy admitted. "After the bad relationship, I was thinking of becoming the first Protestant nun."

"That would have been a big loss," Gabe said spontaneously. "You have all these great wife skills."

She blushed in response and sent Gabe a message to proceed more slowly when she changed the subject. "I'll bet you can give me the scientific name for everything in this meal."

"I could, but the scientific mood isn't on me." He poured more tea into her cup.

"So how did you get your grandmother's house?" she asked.

"My grandparents left it to my mother, and she left it to me. All the property on the reservation belongs to the tribe so it has to pass through a family. If a family is left without an heir, the property goes back to the tribe. I had good memories of visiting here so I've kept it like it was when I was a kid. Not much like the usual bachelor apartment, is it?"

"You're not like the usual bachelor." She paused. "For example, you're the first guy I've known who likes hot tea. I might have thought you made it for me, but you didn't know it's my favorite thing to drink."

"I got hooked on it in graduate school. My mentor was from England, and if you went to his office to talk you were going to get hot tea. Now it's my favorite thing to drink, and I'm the only person I know who likes it hot. Dr. George used to tell me you didn't dare go to England and ask for iced tea. There are some places in the south where they give you a look if you ask for it hot."

Christy held the cup in her hands and remembered her grandmother. "My grandma used to make it for me every night. She had an old tin teapot with an infuser inside it." She smiled at Gabe and said, "I have a really weird request."

"I can't wait to hear it." Gabe saw her blush and wondered what she would ask.

"Can I see your uniform?" she asked tentatively.

"I don't know." Gabe grinned. "I don't usually show it to girls on the first date, but then this date is really special." He stood. "It would be a pleasure to show it to you, Miss Fielding." He left her in the living room and returned with two uniforms, one white and one blue. "These were my dress uniforms. The Navy gives you a selection. I have a lot of other uniforms, but I thought these must be what you wanted to see. Now I get to ask why."

Christy blushed again as she came over and examined the white uniform. "There was this old movie I was absolutely nuts about when I was thirteen. The guy had this kind of uniform."

"I'll bet that was *An Officer and a Gentleman*. Do you know I had girls ask me out because of that movie?" His eyes asked the question, and she read his face easily.

"That wasn't why I wanted to go out with you. I didn't know you were in the Navy until tonight. I just liked you. It was like I already knew you. My friend at the store, Joannie, likes you, too." She looked up at him with crystalline blue eyes. "I thought you should know because she's a lot prettier than I am."

"Not to me," Gabe said. At that moment, he knew he hadn't ever seen a more attractive girl. Looking into her eyes mesmerized him. "Your eyes are the same color as the Caribbean Sea," he said. "I'll bet no other guy ever said that to you." Christy laughed and shook her head.

"No one ever said that. I would remember if they had." She examined his uniform again and realized he had several medals and even more ribbons. One medal was a silver star, and she pointed to it.

"What's this for?"

"It's a medal for getting hurt while trying to rescue someone else. That's what I got before I took medical discharge." He put the uniforms across the sofa carefully. "You wouldn't have gotten the dress whites thrill if I hadn't been an officer."

"I was almost sure you had been. I could tell by the way you led your troops. I see your uniforms get tender loving care," she teased him.

"The Navy pounds that rule into your head early on. The uniform reflects on you and the service. If a sailor is stupid enough to show up in a dirty or wrinkled uniform once, he definitely won't forget a second time. What else do you want to see?"

"Everything about you," she said. His smile was her reward. The words were impulsive, but Christy had made the decision to really know Gabe Killian. She was sure he was worth the risk.

CHAPTER 4

They returned to the kitchen and washed the few dishes while Gabe thought of how he could prolong their time together. As Christy wiped the last plate, he asked, "So when do you want to start your martial arts lessons?"

"How about tonight?" The answer was confirmation that she wanted more time with him.

Gabe opened the back door and turned on the eaves lights. "This is a better place to teach you. There's more room. I need you to take off your shoes."

"Why?" she asked in bewilderment.

"Because I'm the one you're going to be hitting." She sat down and removed her tennis shoes and socks, watching as he removed his sport sandals.

"So this is going to be a serious contact sport?" she said dubiously.

"Well, I certainly hope so." Gabe grinned. "You'll have to hit me to learn how to hit. I just get to grab you."

"Oh." Her eyes were wide as he took her hand and led her into the middle of the yard. He stepped behind her and put his arms around her waist loosely.

"OK. For you, running is the best tactic. I've seen you run. If you can get a head start, they aren't likely to catch you. So you've been grabbed from behind, and you've got to get your attacker to let go. You need three blows to distract them." He paused. "Change places so I can show you."

Christy moved around him and put her arms around his waist. He looked over his shoulder and said, "This is definitely better."

She couldn't help but laugh. He showed her the moves without hurting her. Then they changed places again, and he made her hit him to make certain she understood. As she became more confident in the moves, she began to hit him with more strength. She couldn't feel any reaction to her blows but understood that was due to his strength and not any problem with her technique. By ten o'clock she had learned some basic blocks and three blows.

"I guess I should get you to take me home," Christy said reluctantly. "I know it's getting late, but I kind of wanted to see you do some martial arts."

"I'll be happy to show off because watching will keep you here that much longer. I'd always heard about time flying, but I didn't believe it could until tonight." He pointed to the back steps and said, "Take a seat." He did a black belt kata, losing himself in the art form as he always did.

Christy couldn't take his eyes off him. Though he was performing an Asian form of martial arts, her artist's mind saw him as a warrior. As she watched him, she realized everything about him fascinated her. When he finished, she applauded loudly.

"You're really good. How long have you been studying martial arts?"

"Since I was a kid. When I was in graduate school, I still went to some of the tournaments, but I haven't had time since I started teaching. I practice to stay in shape.

I have one of those store everything metabolisms that would have me suffering from dunlap's disease if I ever stopped exercising."

"Dunlap's disease?" Christy asked.

"Where your belly done lapped over your belt." He laughed at her expression. "Look around you. Obesity and diabetes are an epidemic in this country. There's nothing I want to eat so much that I'm willing to die for it. I remember my mother saying food was the only pleasure she had left. That's a sickness more than diabetes is."

He took her hand and led her to the back door, drawing her into his arms slowly. She felt a tremendous sense of anticipation before he actually kissed her. When his mouth touched hers, she was overwhelmed by the sensation. She had been kissed by other men, but she had never felt such a wave of desire from just one kiss. His hands on her back pressed her gently forward until their bodies were clasped together. Her hands slipped from his shoulders to his arms, and she clung to him as they continued the kiss. Their bodies were so close that she could feel his heart rate accelerate to match her own. She was looking up into his eyes when he released her, and she had the feeling she could trust him with her life. They both stood very still just looking at each other for several moments while their bodies urged them to continue the moment. The second kiss was even more provocative. Christy felt as if Gabe Killian could read exactly how she was feeling. She exhaled in a shuddering breath when he released her.

"I promised myself to always be honest from the beginning of any relationship, Gabe," she said as much for herself as for him. "I don't believe in sleeping around. I never have."

"Neither do I," he promised. "When I got back from the Navy, I became a Christian. Living like one is my top priority. I can already tell that's going to be a challenge when I'm with you." The words made her smile and realize she wanted and needed to be attractive to him.

They sat down to put on their shoes. He took her hand and led her through the house. He stopped only to lock the back door and turn off the kitchen lights. As they left the house, Christy found herself wishing she didn't have to leave Gabe Killian. In the truck, she moved to the middle seat and put on that seat belt.

"I'm a Christian, too," she said. "I know what you mean about feeling tempted. I didn't know until tonight." His smile told her they were on the same wavelength, and he drove back to Bryson City with his arm around her.

"Why did you leave the Navy?" she asked as they drove down the interstate.

"I got hurt really bad. My Seal team was doing reconnaissance in a not-so-friendly country, and when we got back to our extraction point we were ambushed. When they drop Seals off for a mission, it's called the insertion, and the departure is called an extraction. It's not easy to get out when you're under fire. We call that a hot extraction, and we have drills to teach us to handle it.

"Unfortunately, the drills don't prepare you for everything that can happen. I got shot in my shoulder and fell off the dock. The beach was rocky. I didn't remember anything except falling until a month later. I fractured my skull, and because of the bleeding from the fracture I lost most of the peripheral vision in my left eye. That isn't the kind of disability that lends itself to a special forces career.

"I knew I'd end up behind a desk somewhere, so I took a medical discharge. It wasn't easy. I had been in the Navy my whole adult life. I had wanted to serve until I retired. While I was wallowing in self pity, my uncle came to visit me and he said, 'You know, Gabe, you can't expect life to treat you any better than Jesus was treated. So if you haven't been crucified because you were God's son, you really don't have any right to complain.' I hadn't ever thought of it that way, but he's right."

"So you can't see on the left?" she asked. "Does it bother you?"

"It did, but not any more. I focus on listening and feeling the air move on that side of my face. It's not easy for anyone to surprise me now. I guess that sounds sort of paranoid, but I had to live that way when I was a Seal. My life depended on not letting anyone surprise me. I know I'm lucky to be able to complain about it. The residual damage could have been a whole lot worse. When I first woke up, I couldn't see well at all. What I could see was just outlines and shadows. My balance was gone. If I stood up, I fell down. I was so dizzy I couldn't eat without getting sick. The neurologists weren't sure whether it would go away or not. They were afraid I was going to have a seizure disorder because of the damage.

"I don't usually take medicine, but I was on all sorts of drugs to keep me together. Gradually it started resolving, which is proof God knew how much I could stand. The only thing I'm aware of now is the peripheral vision being gone." He took her hand and put it on the back of his head. She could feel the faint outline of a very large scar under his hair. "Fortunately my hair is long enough to cover the souvenir."

There was a moment of silence, and then Christy asked the question she needed to ask.

"Were you ever married, Gabe?"

"No. I haven't even been close," he said. "I'll have to make it forever when I get married." He picked up her left hand. "How about you?"

She shook her head and then pointed at a narrow winding road going up the mountain.

"It's hard to turn around ahead," she said. "I'll walk the rest of the way." She waited until he had stopped the truck and then turned to kiss him. From the moment he put his arms around her, she lost herself in the kiss. She was breathless when he released her and knew he didn't really want to stop either. She had to force herself to slide across the seat and out the door. Then she stood looking at him and wanting to get back into the truck.

"The time really did fly."

"How about a phone number, Christy?" His voice was almost pleading.

"If I had a phone, I'd give the number to you. I have a low standard of living these days." She reached out for his hand. "I do want to see you again if the drive isn't too far."

"It would have to be a whole lot farther to keep me away. I might come around tomorrow afternoon if that isn't too soon."

"I'd like for you to come around tomorrow." Her eyes glowed softly in the moonlight. "I had a great time, Gabe."

He watched her walk up the dirt road until she disappeared into the darkness. He drove home slowly, thinking of her all the way there. He had never missed anyone's company as much as he missed Christy. He felt inconsolably alone.

He put away his uniforms and returned to the living room looking for a way to pass the time. When Job arrived at midnight, Gabe was sitting cross-legged on the floor listening to a Native American flute ensemble and flipping through photograph albums at the pictures of his childhood in Jonah and Reba's home. He hadn't felt he had a home since leaving them at the age of sixteen.

Job plopped down on the floor and looked over his shoulder. "The retrospective mode?"

"I guess you could say that," Gabe said. "You decide about what future you want based on what you like in your past. We were really lucky to have your parents." He closed the book. "Did you and Darla have a good time?"

"A most excellent adventure," Job said. He studied Gabe's face. "You went out, too. We drove by at ten o'clock and your truck wasn't here."

"Well, I'm not too old to go out, you know." Gabe closed the photo album with finality. "I think I've met my soul mate, Job. Pray about it for me because I've either lost my mind or finally found it. I drove home thinking about marriage after one date."

"Wow. You need to talk to dad. That's a little too deep for me."

"Just add it to your prayer list," Gabe said good-natured voice. "I'm not planning to elope. Just thinking about what it would be like to have a wife and kids. It's pretty cool actually because I've never had those thoughts before."

Gabe's alarm clock was turned off on Saturdays, but he awakened abruptly at seven o'clock and packed to spend a day in the woods. He was at Deep Creek just as a crowd of summer revelers began arriving at the convenience store. Christy was surrounded and harassed, but she smiled at him and waved as he set out on his hike. It was a good day for field biology. He located two species of wildflowers that were endangered. He photographed both and carefully documented their location. He didn't return to the station until almost six o'clock; he had already stood under two waterfalls to cool off.

"You're so lucky," Christy commented. He was still dripping in mute testimony to his swim. "I'd have given a million bucks to be in the creek at three this afternoon. At least I brought clothes so I can change this time."

"I can wait for you while you shower here or we can go to my place. Your choice." He glanced at the huge disarray of inner tubes and continued, "Will your boss be upset if I help you out?"

"Only if you charge him for it," Christy said. "I'd appreciate it. I hate Saturdays."

"I'm driven to make them better days for you." Gabe locked his gear in his truck and returned to help her bring order from chaos. When they finished, they were both soaked in sweat and smeared with mud.

"Waterfall time," Christy said and punctuated the idea by running up the trail. Gabe pursued her but allowed her to win the one mile race to the larger Indian Creek Falls. When she hesitated to climb down, Gabe passed her and dove into the water without hesitation. Christy jumped in feet first and surfaced just below the falls, still trying to catch her breath. Gabe popped up beside her.

"Cold water on a hot day is an extreme high," Christy sighed. "You really shouldn't dive into the water when you don't know how deep it is."

"I've been diving into this pool since I was nine," Gabe reassured her. "This time of year, it's fifteen feet in the center. We used to slide down the falls, but that really isn't safe. There are too many hidden rocks you can hit."

Christy swam over to the shallows and stood in the chest deep water. "You jumped into it from ten feet up the bank. That's a big drop."

"Not when you've jumped into the ocean from an airplane." Gabe laughed at her expression. "To avoid radar, sometimes they made us parachute out of commercial air space. Before that, I didn't really love heights. I was desensitized the first day they dropped us off at 30,000 feet."

"Are you trying to shock me?"

"I'm trying to impress you. Trying to impress the pretty girl is essential during 'getting to know you' dates." He dove under the surface again and came up shaking the water from his hair. "Finish cooling off, and let's head for Qualla Boundary."

The moon was just rising when they hiked down the mountain trail to the campground. Gabe unlocked the truck while Christy retrieved her backpack. When she climbed into the truck beside him, she asked, "What's Qualla Boundary?"

"It's the land that belongs to the Cherokee tribe. Otherwise known as the reservation." Gabe started the engine and said, "I was thinking you could stay the night with my aunt and uncle and go to church with me tomorrow. No pressure. It's just a thought."

"I'm supposed to work, but where else will Bo get slave labor if he fires me? Are you sure they won't mind? I could sleep in a sleeping bag in your back yard."

"Cherokee is a small town. Your reputation could be messed up if you spent the night at my place. Reba and Jonah are really nice. They won't mind."

Christy reached out to take his hand, feeling pleasure when his fingers curled around hers. She could feel the strength in his hands and the gentleness he wanted her to feel.

"If they really wouldn't mind, I'd like to stay. I haven't had any good times since my grandmother died. Yesterday was the first day I've enjoyed in a long time."

He stopped at a traffic light and pulled her close to kiss her as if they were high school sweethearts. Cars honked to get them going again, but it didn't matter. Christy was glad to move closer to him and feel his arm around her shoulders. Even the silences between them were comfortable.

CHAPTER 5

Before Gabe and Christy reached Cherokee, she started telling him about herself. It didn't seem a risk because she was sure she could trust him. She was surprised to learn they shared the same birthday, September 1, with ten years between them.

"At least I know you're old enough to date," he teased her. He pulled into his driveway and opened the truck door for her before unlocking the house door. He gave her first access to the bathroom and made them both a glass of iced tea while she was getting changed. Then he called Jonah and asked for the favor he had already offered.

When Christy reappeared in a sea green sun dress with her hair loose on her shoulders, he whistled admiringly.

"Sorry for the macho demonstration, but you look great."

"Every girl likes that kind of macho," she replied. "I was kind of hoping you'd like this dress." She couldn't tell him that she had bought it on her lunch hour that day to impress him.

"You're a terrific success," he said. "I'll be right out." While he was gone, she moved around the living room and dining room of the house recognizing that some of the pictures were clearly Gabe's and not a part of his inheritance. The one over the mantle drew her attention because it was a photograph of the mountains taken at Newfound Gap. The photographer had caught the wafting mist sliding through the blue peaks. A series of characters was inscribed on the inner mat. The same sort of characters were on a framed eagle feather over an old mahogany bookcase. All the artwork was of the Smoky Mountains. She was staring at the characters under the photograph when Gabe returned and stood behind her.

"I'll bet you're wondering what it says," he said.

"You win," she replied. "What does it say?"

"Psalms 121," Gabe said. "'I will lift up my eyes unto the hills from whence cometh my help.' That's my favorite Psalm. I think everyone I know on the reservation feels like we draw some special source of strength from these 'hills.' I took that picture, and after it was matted, I painted the verse on the mat in Cherokee."

"You're a good photographer," Christy said in admiration.

"I hate to lower your opinion of me, but I took about two hundred shots before I got that one. Fortunately I'm computer literate and did them digitally, or I'd be sacking groceries to pay for the film."

Christy pointed to the eagle feather. "What's the significance of that one?"

"That's an award from the tribe for being a veteran. They gave it to me when I came home. Eagles are sacred to most Native American people. The legends say they don't die. Their spirits move on even if their body is destroyed. To get an eagle feather is a big honor. Only Native Americans can own eagle feathers without getting into trouble with the Department of the Interior."

"What do the characters say?" She glanced back when he took a moment to answer.

"Gabriel Killian, Cherokee warrior. It means a lot to me. Probably more than anything else in this house." Christy turned to look at him, reading how serious he was in his eyes.

"That's because it's a way of life and not just a title," she said. Gabe looked surprised that she understood.

"The right way of doing things." He was wearing a shirt decorated in earth tones that were unmistakably Native American.

"Was your shirt made in Cherokee?" Christy asked.

"It's Navajo made," he said. "I got it on the Navajo reservation when I was stationed out west. The Seal training facility is in San Diego. After they finish torturing you for twenty-five weeks, you get leave to vent. I'd never considered myself to be a quitter, but there were times when I wanted to walk off from the Seal training. They call part of it 'hell week,' if that tells you anything. When I made it through, it was an eagle feather moment. Then I had a pressing need to be alone in the wilderness, so I went to Mesa Verde in New Mexico to climb the cliffs." He took her hand and led her to the truck while continuing to tell her about that part of his life.

"There are ruins in the cliffs from hundreds of years ago. They were made by a tribe called the Anasazi. It was like stepping back in time. You can't believe the climb those people made every day. The rocks had perfectly spaced hand and toe holds. When you get to the top, there's a fortress still perfectly preserved after eight hundred years.

"They call the desert there big sky country. At night you can see just about every star in the northern hemisphere. One night when I was camping, I watched a meteor shower. After that I almost decided to go to flight school. A lot of the astronauts are Navy pilots, and I gave thought to being the first Cherokee astronaut."

Christy was so mesmerized that she forgot to be hungry as they drove to the reservation's casino parking lot.

"What changed your mind?"

"I had to be an officer first. That meant I had to graduate from college. When I had my degree in biology, I realized I really loved being a diver. The ocean is a lot like space. We haven't explored very much of it, and the deeper we go the more we find out we don't know. I've done some submarine work, and I spent all my free time with my nose pasted to the portholes like a kid looking in a toy store."

"I don't think I'd like being enclosed like that," Christy shuddered. "How did you stand it?"

"Looking out the window," Gabe admitted. "I hate being enclosed, but when they let us out, being in the ocean felt like coming home." He was silent for a long moment. Christy felt his emotions as clearly as if he had voiced them.

"You still miss it."

"Sometimes," Gabe said. "I love these mountains as much or more than the sea. As time has passed, I've come to know that I'm a part of this place, and it's a part of me. The scenery has gotten even better in the last few days." Christy blushed and smiled in response to his compliment.

"So what was your rank?" she asked.

"I was a lieutenant commander when I was discharged." He cut off the ignition and took her hand. "Let's have supper. We can still talk in the restaurant."

Christy was wide eyed as they entered the restaurant.

"This is definitely the nicest restaurant I've ever been to."

"It's a big money maker," Gabe said. "The reservation has needed a better financial support system for a long time. Actually it's sort of a movement all over America because gambling is legal on reservations. The money goes back into the tribal coffers to improve education and health care. I don't believe in gambling myself, but it's good to see some good come out of it. When I was a kid, this was a poor town. People had to live off the tourist season. Some of it was pretty degrading. There are people who still believe the Cherokee wore big feather war bonnets."

"And you don't?" Christy teased him.

"Originally the Cherokee men wore two feathers tied into their scalp lock. The rest of their hair was shaved. After the settlers came, they wore turbans. The war bonnets are for the tourists. Some of them get their whole concept of what it is to be an Indian from grade B movies." His voice was teasing, but Christy knew he was very serious about his heritage.

"I don't have any preconceived notions," she said as she smiled. "I'm sorry I interrupted you. Go on."

"Back then, unemployment was rampant, and a lot of people survived only because of government subsidy. With nothing to bring us pride, alcoholism was a big problem. The only thing that protected us was the law Chief Drowning Bear made back in the 1800s making the Qualla Boundary alcohol free. Even the casino is dry. If you want to drink, you'll have to buy it elsewhere and bring it back. Now everyone who teaches here tries to make the kids understand we're genetically susceptible to alcoholism, so it's a good idea not to ever try it. I can see that personally because I tried drinking when I was in the Navy, and it's very seductive. You can drown whatever is bothering you with a certain number of drinks. Jonah made me see that's a message from God to stop while you can."

They ordered, and Christy felt embarrassed when she realized she had ordered twice as much food as Gabe had. He had a large salad with the dressing on the side. She felt very self conscious when the waitress brought their suppers. Gabe didn't seem to notice.

"You're really serious about your diet, aren't you?" she said as she dug into her plate.

"Totally. If I eat much at night, I have to run for about three hours to burn it off. Too much of my job is sedentary now. I've gained about fifteen pounds since I left the service because I'm sitting so much more than I used to. You're one of those incredibly blessed people who can eat anything and not gain weight, aren't you?"

Christy blushed. "I don't eat like this very often. I haven't eaten like this in years."

"Don't feel guilty about good metabolism. I want this to be a special night for you. Maybe not because of the food, but I'll take what I can get."

"The food is a really small part of the special feeling."

They talked all through their meal, never losing interest in each other. Christy had never met a man who made her feel so at ease. During that hour, she forgot to be afraid. Gabe had a second cup of tea while she ate a piece of cheesecake. Too soon they were finished eating and didn't have an excuse to stay longer. Christy wondered if the date could be the beginning of a new life.

"Will anybody give you a hard time about dating me, Gabe?" she asked anxiously. "I don't have much to bring into a relationship."

"I can't say that I care what anybody thinks," he said. "I'm actually looking for a whole lot more than a dowry." He gave his credit card to the waitress. "My friends will probably be relieved. I don't go out that much. I've been waiting for the right girl to come along, and here you are."

She felt a rush of joy. "I haven't gone out with any-body in a long time either. Now I'm getting swept off my feet."

He took her hand and held it between both of his hands. "Now you're rewarding me with positive feed-back like you got for how you look tonight. I was hoping for that kind of success."

She wanted to kiss him across the candle-lit table and instead found herself staring into his eyes as if all the answers she had been waiting for were in him. The waitress interrupted them by placing the check beside Gabe's left elbow. He looked up as if surprised and then signed the check.

"I didn't even hear her coming. You're incredibly dis-tracting, Christy." They both smiled, and Gabe said, "The evening's young. Where do you want to go next?"

"I thought I saw a carnival down the road. I haven't been on a roller coaster since I was a little girl."

They rode every ride in the little amusement park, finishing on a ferris wheel. When they were at the top, the wheel stopped to allow other people to get off. Christy leaned back against Gabe's arm and looked up into his dark eyes. She knew she was falling in love because she couldn't keep her eyes off him. She didn't like heights, but Gabe made her feel safe even a hundred feet off the ground.

"What are you thinking?" he asked.

"How you make me feel," she said softly. "I've never felt like you make me feel." She put her hand on his face very gently and closed her eyes as he pulled her even closer. His hands ran through her hair and then closed over the thick mass. He kissed her as they sat on top of the ride and kept kissing her until all she could feel was his mouth and his arms. All she could hear was the blood rushing in her ears. The feeling was overpowering for her and for Gabe. Neither of them had any desire to stop.

They were so involved in feeling each other that they didn't realize the ferris wheel had brought them to the exit. The operator laughed and sent them around again. At the top, with her hand on his chest over his heart, Christy whispered, "I'm falling in love with you, Gabe, and I don't think I could handle having my heart broken again."

"I've been feeling the same way," Gabe said. "I promise you don't need to be afraid of being with me. I couldn't ever hurt you. I know how it feels to be betrayed by someone you love." He intended to just kiss her lightly, but he lost himself in the feeling of holding her. They made three more trips around before they could bring themselves to get off. It was almost midnight when Gabe drove Christy to his uncle's house, fighting the urge to park on numerous dark streets. He pulled her into his arms for one last embrace in his uncle's driveway and then led her to the front door. Jonah answered his knock and smiled at the two.

"You must be Christy. I'm Jonah Killian. My wife is making our guest room ready. We'll see you in the morning, Gabe."

"Thanks, Jonah," Gabe said. "You'll never know how much I appreciate this."

"I'll save the return favor for the future," Jonah said.

Christy looked back at Gabe as Jonah escorted her into his house. Gabe stood outside for several minutes more wishing he could take her home with him and make his home *their* home. As he drove to his house, he spent his time trying to decide how little time he could know Christy and marry her. He was certain the haste he wanted would elicit a flurry of protestations from his family and friends. For the first time in his adult life, he didn't really care what anyone else thought.

CHAPTER 6

Christy lay awake a long time thinking of Gabe. She knew slowing down the torrent of their emotional relationship would probably be a good idea. Nonetheless, she had no desire to hold anything back. She had believed she would always be in danger from the Divilbiss family. That night she told herself that after twenty-one months they must have forgotten someone as insignificant as she was. She thought of Gabe's military experience and how he had offered to protect her. She had heard that the special forces in the military were much better trained than most police officers. Still, she didn't think he could take the threat against her seriously until she told him more. She was afraid to tell him more for fear of losing him. Then she thought of how pointless her existence had been for such a long time. Even if it was a risk to tell Gabe Killian her story, it seemed like her only chance to take control of her destiny again.

As if God were affirming her decision, she had the best day of her life that Sunday. Jonah Killian's church was the sort of family church where even strangers could feel at home. Christy was greeted by so many people that she briefly lost Gabe at the end of the service. Reba took her to the Sunday school class of high school students he taught. She entered quietly and took a seat in the back of the room. The question Gabe was answering later seemed prophetic. At that moment, Christy took his answer very personally.

"The whole idea behind the book of Job is that what happens in this life has nothing to do with how good or bad a person is. Evil happens to very good people. Tragedies occur. What God wants from us is to believe He'll let us find the strength and courage to deal with whatever happens to us. Accepting difficulties can make us witnesses to God's support. Sometimes I think the lesson from when the Israelites wandered forty years in the wilderness is that we shouldn't have any goal greater than following God. We might be better off if we just keep our eyes on the cloud even if we aren't sure where it's going to take us." He smiled in Christy's direction as he responded to the next question. He couldn't know that she felt as if he had been directed to give those words to her.

They lingered at the church until everyone else had left and then had dinner with Gabe's family. She got to meet Job's sister, Naomi, who was a teacher at the elementary school. Her husband, Eddie Owle, ran a white-water rafting outfit on the local rivers.

Christy was treated as if she was already Gabe's wife. No one showed any signs that she was different because she wasn't a Native American. It was obvious that his family was very fond of Gabe and proud of his accomplishments, and all of them took a turn at bragging.

"He was the second Killian to graduate from college," Jonah informed her. "No one had gone beyond high school until I went to Bible college. I think Gabriel surprised himself. He never liked school before the Navy."

"I was a low man on the Navy totem pole when I realized the advantages of officer's candidate school," Gabe said. "I'd already been to the warrant officer's training, but you can't go beyond warrant officer if you don't have a degree so I decided I wanted a degree. They gave me all the basic classes and then asked me what I wanted my major to be. I remember making a smart remark about majoring in ocean life. Next thing I knew I was registered as a biology major. I never expected to like it. At first, I took some unmerciful kidding about it from the other Seals. The other officers had their degrees in political science or sociology. I was already taking a lot of grief since I was a chief petty officer or in Navy lingo I was Chief Killian. I was about ready to deck the next idiot that left a feather on my bunk. When I was studying sea life, they got off their 'haze the Indian' mission and started asking me questions. When I had to figure out how to answer them, I learned more. I got into the teacher mode then."

"Tell her about your dissertation," Job urged Gabe. "He studied these bacteria that live in geysers and the super deep places in the ocean. It's like sci-fi but for real."

"I have friends that are working in oceanography in the Navy, and they had access to samples from the vents. The vents are like geysers on the bottom of the ocean. It's not as big of a deal as Job makes it out to be."

"He was offered a position at the big oceanography institute in Florida," Job bragged. "They take only one new scientist every three years."

"Don't build me up too much, Job. She won't believe any of it if you keep exaggerating."

Gabe pulled Christy aside after lunch and suggested that they needed to leave if they wanted to go hiking. They both thanked Jonah and Reba before their departure. While Christy was talking to Reba, Gabe went to say good-bye to Job, Eddie, and Naomi. When Christy came to join him, she realized they were speaking a language she didn't understand. When she and Gabe were in his truck, she asked him about it.

"What were you saying to your cousins?"

"What was I saying? Oh. We were speaking Cherokee. Our language is written and spoken, and it's required in the schools here now. It was almost a lost language forty years ago so we're all obsessed with keeping it alive. Especially Naomi. That's her passion. I'll teach you." He grinned. "It's impossible to keep a teacher from teaching."

They changed into shorts and tee shirts at Gabe's house. Then, he drove her up to the continental divide.

"You made a great impression," he told her. "Jonah and Job both gave you the two thumbs-up sign. I told you they would be glad to see me going out with you. I'm setting the record for the oldest bachelor in Killian history. My grandfather held the previous record. He got married when he was thirty, but that wasn't the same because my grandmother was his second wife. His first wife died, and he stayed single for seven years."

"You're so lucky," Christy said slowly. "I only had my grandmother until she died. I always wished for a big family."

"They're a tremendous blessing. Jonah especially." Gabe glanced at her. "My stepfather was very abusive. He put a permanent wedge between me and my mother. If I hadn't had Jonah and Reba, I probably would have self destructed. I was headed that way when I joined the Navy. Joining was sort of a way to run away from my problems. The first year I tried smoking, drinking, swearing, and just about everything else I'd ever been told not to do. I was really angry then. I got to be a better runner because that was our basic training instructor's favorite punishment. Sometimes I have a hard time remembering how many years it's been since I was your age.

"I can't forget how it was when I first got back from the Navy. Jonah and Reba took care of me while I was recovering. I had a really hard time dealing with it for the first six months. Jonah prayed with me every day even when I didn't believe God was listening."

"What made you believe?" Christy asked. He hesitated for several moments as he parked the truck and turned off the ignition.

"You may think I'm completely nuts when I tell you this. I guess that means it's a real relationship test." He leaned on his elbow. "I didn't want to feel dependent on anyone including God for most of my life. Jonah was chipping away at that issue while I was trying to decide where I was going with my life after the Navy. He kept telling me to pray for a sign. Finally I did. It was after he gave me his famous 'you don't have a right to complain' speech. I didn't really believe I'd get an answer, but I prayed. That night, I dreamed about my father. I've seen his pictures, Christy, but he died when I was a baby. He saw me once when I was two weeks old. I don't have any memory of him at all, but I saw him in my dream. He sat down and told me what he had wanted to do with his life.

"When I woke up, it felt like it had really happened. I remembered everything he had said, but I thought I was making too much of it. I finally asked Jonah about my father and what his dreams had been. He brought out this box he had saved after my grandparents died. Everything in that box related to what was in my dream. I knew God had given that knowledge to me. I knew I hadn't died for a reason. Everything came together. How could I deny what was in front of me? I was baptized a week later. After that, it's been easy to pray. I pray all the time, and it keeps me focused more than anything else." He took her hand. "Come with me. I want to show you something."

They hiked to chimney tops and Klingman's Dome. Gabe showed her the dying evergreens.

"Acid rain did this. It's killing more of the plant life all the time. I've been pulling these samples on my own trying to work on what makes them vulnerable. I dream of finding a way to protect the plants from what we've done to the atmosphere. Big dream, isn't it?"

"That's why you didn't go to that institute, isn't it?" she said.

"That's why." He was surprised that she could know something he hadn't even shared with his family. "I believe everything happens for a reason. Maybe I'm meant to be a conservationist. That's why I took the survey job with the park service."

"That was what your father wanted to do." Christy knew she had surmised correctly by Gabe's expression. She was startled by her own clairvoyance. She had never been able to read someone so easily.

"My father wanted to be a forest ranger and learn how to protect the land," Gabe said. "He had filled out a college application to UNC to study biology. He had a packet of information on how to join the Park Ranger program. Jonah said he was always interested in bringing nature back into balance. In high school he wrote papers on recycling before anyone considered it feasible. I had worked on any recycling project I could find when I was in high school. I never knew my father had felt the same way until the dream. Native Americans have always believed dreams were powerful messages from God." He looked at her intently. "Have you always had ESP?"

"I don't have it. At least I don't think I do." She smiled and put her hand on his arm. "I feel like we're connected, Gabe. It's like I've known you for a long time. It's a weird feeling, but it's kind of comforting, too."

"I've never felt connected to anyone like I feel with you," he admitted. He took her hand and made her turn to face him. "Now I'm wondering if God had a two-part answer to my prayer."

The light coming over his shoulders seemed to illuminate his face. The vision made Christy think of the picture of the angel Gabriel in her Bible. She allowed herself to think that Gabriel Killian was like an angel sent to deliver her from evil. She slipped into his arms and held him tightly for several moments, feeling safe and secure as he held her.

"Maybe you're the answer to my prayers."

They returned to the parking lot by an unmarked and minimally populated trail, stopping at a creek to cool off when the afternoon heat made them sweat. They stretched out on the bank to lie in the filtered sun holding hands.

"So what do you dream about?" Gabe asked her.

"I wanted to be an artist. All I've been able to dream about for the last year is surviving on my own." She smiled and shrugged. "Someday." He leaned over her and kissed her.

"Someday doesn't have to be so far away, Christy. For me, it's looking closer all the time. You never finished your degree, did you?"

"I had to get away." She looked away from him as the memory of Chuck's death returned in a rush. The memory made her terrified for Gabe Killian. She knew he would be at risk if she allowed him to remain in her life, and she regretted letting him get so close to her. She made a wane effort to put some distance between them.

"The other person in the relationship wanted to hurt me, and I think he still would if he could find me." Gabe turned her face toward him very gently as he recognized her fear. He knew it was standing between them, and he felt afraid of anything that could come between them.

"I can protect you, Christy. I won't let him hurt you. I'm probably better equipped to protect you than anyone else you know." He caressed her hair. "You could enroll at the college where I teach, and you'd be close to me all day. You could move closer so we could be together almost all the time." He stopped abruptly as he started to ask her to move in with him. He sat up slowly knowing it was wrong to even have the thought. In the same moment, he knew he wanted to marry her. He spoke his only reservation without realizing he was speaking aloud. "I never believed in the idea of people falling in love in just a matter of days. Biologists say it's just some sort of hormonal reaction, but it isn't."

Christy sat up and put her hands on his shoulders feeling the need to accept what he had almost offered. On impulse she kissed his shoulder and then rested her face on his back. "If I didn't care about you, I'd take every one of your suggestions. It wouldn't be fair to you, Gabe. You don't know me." He pulled her into his arms and kissed her as if she were his wife.

"I do know you, Christy. Just like you know me."

They hiked out of the wilderness because they were both feeling a heightened need for their relationship to go faster and farther than they knew it should. They spent the end of the day sitting in Gabe's back yard watching the stars come out. He brought out a telescope and showed her the rings around Saturn and the craters on the moon.

"How did you become an astronomer?" she asked as she scanned the moon's surface.

"I was always drawn to the stars. When I was at sea, I'd stand on the deck at night and watch the stars come out. You know it's all different in the southern hemisphere." He lay back with his head on his folded arms and watched her explore the heavens. After a while, she lay back with her head on his shoulder. He closed his arm around her and pulled her even closer. He wasn't feeling any need to make love at that moment. It felt comforting just to hold her.

"It feels good," she murmured.

"What does?" he asked although he knew what her answer would be.

"Being close to you. I wish I could stay here with you." Christy sighed and closed her eyes hoping she could just sleep beside him on the grass in his back yard. She felt both safe and content.

For a long time Gabe held her and thought of just sleeping on the grass with her in his arms. When Job returned home, appearances made him awaken her. It was just before midnight. They started the drive to Bryson City reluctantly. It was a silent ride for much of the way because both of them were lost in their thoughts. When they stopped at the path to Christy's home, she clung to Gabe. She knew she should tell him she wouldn't be free at least until the weekend. She thought if she didn't see him, she would die.

"Tomorrow seems a long way off," she whispered. "I know I'll only be able to stand waiting for the time to pass if I know I'll see you again."

"You will. I promise you will." He kissed her until he had to make himself let her go. "This is one of those times I'm praying really hard to get past temptation. I don't want to leave you here. I'm going to talk to Jonah and Reba. Maybe you could live with them for a little while."

She trembled with the need to accept his unspoken offer. She wanted to ask him to take her home because his house already felt like the only port in the storm of her life.

"I have to go, Gabriel," she said. The way her voice caressed his name gave Gabe a physical thrill. He had never been called Gabriel, but he had wanted to earn the honor of using his grandfather's name. She made him feel as if the name were finally his own.

He kissed her and held her again. "I don't want to let you go."

"If I don't go, I might stay," she whispered. "I want to stay even when I know it would be wrong." She extricated herself from his arms and got out of the truck. She walked to his side to kiss him. "Thank you for being with me. You're the only good time I can remember having." She released his hand and began the long walk up the mountainside hoping he would follow her and praying he wouldn't. When she heard the truck door open, she turned to meet him.

"At least let me walk you home," Gabe said. "It's too dark for you to be climbing this hill all alone."

"I can't, Gabriel," she said. "I might make you stay. You can watch me until I'm out of your sight, and then I'll be home." Gabe hesitated for a long moment and then nodded reluctantly.

"I'll see you tomorrow."

She drifted up the hillside lost in her thoughts. She had to fight the urge to run down the hill and into his arms, and when she was well hidden by the forest, she turned to watch him drive away. All the way home, she kept thinking of Gabriel Killian instead of being pursued. Just when she had given up hope, she felt alive again.

Her bubble burst as she climbed through a maze of kudzu to the place she called home. Kudzu is an imported vine brought to the mountains to prevent the banks from being eroded by the rain. Taking it out of its normal environment has created the equivalent of an Asian jungle in the mountains of the South. It grows down the mountainsides covering everything in its path including trees, buildings, and abandoned vehicles. Kudzu was Christy's protection from discovery and her shield against the weather. That night it was a blessing and a curse. She hadn't ever returned home so late, and the kudzu greatly decreased the moonlight she relied upon to guide her path. As she climbed into her house, she tripped and fell, cutting her leg on an unseen object.

Christy's home was an abandoned school bus on the mountainside. There were other junked cars under the kudzu's heavy foliage, but only the school bus offered shelter from the weather. Christy had survived there even during the winter in conditions only a survivalist could have endured. She had a Coleman stove, a kerosene lantern, a sleeping bag, and a backpack to hold her clothes. That was it. Fresh water was in her canteen. To get more meant a two-mile hike.

Her leg was gashed two inches across, and it bled for a long time. Christy was sure it needed stitches, but that wasn't an option when any registration process would enter her identity into a computer. Chuck's warning had lived in her memory every day since his death. She knew being entered in a computer might make it possible for the Divilbiss family to find her. She washed the cut with the water from her canteen and wrapped it in a tee shirt.

CHAPTER 7

The hike to work made Christy's leg hurt terribly the next morning, and even Bo was alarmed when he saw the redness spreading up from her makeshift bandage. He met her as she came from the campground showers and made her come to his office.

"You should have gone to the emergency room, Christy. This is really deep." He flinched for her as he poured peroxide into the wound and then covered it with gauze. "I can drive you down to the clinic."

"I can't, Bo," Christy said. "Someday I'll tell you why, but now I can't."

She made it through her shift by imagining when Gabe would come. Being without him was almost more painful than her leg. Joannie questioned her about her weekend, and Christy's expression told the tale as much as her words.

"He's unbelievably wonderful, Joannie. He's everything I ever wanted in a guy."

"Does he at least have a brother?" her coworker asked plaintively.

"A cousin, but he's only twenty."

"I can deal with a younger man," Joannie asserted. "At least try to fix me up, Christy."

Christy felt progressively worse as the day passed. She ached and the heat was much more unpleasant than usual. She stuck it out because she believed Gabe would come at six o'clock. She felt like she needed to see him more than she needed to draw her next breath. She stayed long after the others had gone home. It was 6:40 P.M. when she left for home and a walk that had never seemed so long. The message she took home was that Gabe was too busy to see her. She knew she couldn't blame him when she had so little to give a man with everything. He had a home, family, friends, and a career. She had nothing and no one.

She crawled into the bus and lit her lantern long enough to unwrap her leg. The appearance of the wound scared her because the area around the cut was dusky colored. She applied more peroxide and put on a clean bandage using supplies Bo had given her. She counted her blessings for having her tetanus shot up to date and swallowed two anti-inflammatory pills before climbing into her sleeping bag. For the first time she couldn't bring herself to pray for rescue. She didn't feel any motivation to fight for her life because she didn't feel strong enough to keep running and fighting alone. She cried herself to sleep.

Gabe's day had been a frenzy of activity that had robbed him of the chance to meet Christy. It had also been a fall back to earth but for a very different reason. He had been too stirred up by his weekend with Christy to fall asleep until after 2 A.M.. Still he woke up early and was sitting on the porch waiting for the tea to brew and thinking of Christy when Job reminded him he had an appointment at the Veterans Hospital in Asheville.

Gabe had circled the date on the kitchen calendar six months earlier, but uncharacteristically he hadn't looked at the calendar in days. He spent some minutes telling himself that it wasn't all that important. It was a yearly appointment for diabetes screening. Rescheduling it would take three to four months, which he thought wouldn't be a problem. He studied the calendar and noted he would be postponing it to a day during the regular school year. His class schedule through the year made going to Asheville difficult. Keeping the appointment meant a two-hour drive to Asheville, three hours at the hospital, and a two-hour drive back to meet with his only class. He also saw a notation on his calendar that there was a mandatory faculty meeting that afternoon. He said a prayer to get it done, skipped breakfast because he needed to be fasting for the tests and drove to Asheville.

The beginning of the day was deceptively easy. The drive only took an hour and a half. He only had to wait thirty minutes at the clinic to have his blood drawn. The deterioration point came when the doctor came into his exam room.

"I'm Dr. Sawyer, Mr. Killian. We need to talk about your results. I understand you have a very strong family history of diabetes."

"On both sides of my family," Gabe said. Something in the doctor's tone and expression made him uneasy. "Mainly the maternal side. My mother had it. Her brother and both of her parents had it. There were six great uncles and aunts with it. That's why I've wanted to keep up the screening. Most of them had been damaged by the time they knew they had it." The doctor was looking at his chart. Gabe had the feeling that not meeting his gaze was a deliberate act.

"I see you had an episode of steroid induced diabetes when you were injured in the Navy," the doctor continued. "The record said your blood sugar went so high that you needed insulin to control it."

"I don't remember much about the first month after I was injured, but I know I had high blood sugars. They told me that a lot of people have sugar elevations when they get high doses of steroids. I've never had any abnormal blood sugars since then, and I follow a diet and exercise program. I was told that would lower my risk of getting diabetes a lot."

"We're learning more about the development of type 2 diabetes, Mr. Killian. It comes from two problems. One is your inherited tendency to develop insulin resistance. The other is the progressive loss of the cells in your pancreas that make insulin. When people have a high blood sugar after steroids or when women show a high sugar during pregnancy, their bodies are saying that they have already lost enough insulin making cells to have a problem covering their sugar when they are stressed by other hormones. Steroids and the hormones of pregnancy make even normal people resistant to the sugar-lowering effects of insulin. When you have a history of steroid induced diabetes, it usually means your insulin making cells are closer to burning out."

"I understand about the cells burning out," Gabe protested. "That's why diet and exercise are so important to keep blood sugar normal."

"The high sugar is just a symptom of a much bigger disturbance in your metabolism," the doctor said. "We can't just look at sugar because even if you keep your sugar in the normal range, you still have an increased risk of heart disease. When people become diabetic, diet and exercise are not enough to protect them."

"Are you saying that I have it?" Gabe asked in a panic.

Again the doctor refused to meet his gaze. He continued to speak as if his voice could calm a man who believed he was receiving a death sentence. "When your sugar is 126 mg% or higher after not eating for twelve hours, we know your pancreas has failed to compensate for your body's resistance to insulin. The problem is that people are developing damage to their heart and blood vessels years before their sugar starts to go up. There are some people who have fasting blood sugars of less than 126 mg% and still have diabetes if we look at their sugars after meals. Ethnic groups like Native Americans, African Americans, and Hispanic Americans frequently have very high sugars after a sugar load even when their before meal sugars are not high enough to diagnose diabetes. We test for that situation with a glucose tolerance test."

"Please answer my question," Gabe said. "Are you saying I have diabetes?" He knew his voice and his face were expressing his fear. He didn't care. He had put his focus on avoiding the disease and had never let himself think about having it. His next words were a protestation and a denial of what he knew they were going to tell him. "Most of the people in my family were older and overweight when they developed it."

"We're seeing diabetes present at a much younger age now," the doctor said. "We think that's because of the heavy sugar and fat exposure American children get. Most people your age have consumed ten times the amount of sugar their grandparents had consumed by the same age. Diet and exercise can prolong the time until your pancreas fails, but it can't undo what you did by eating too much fat and sugar when you didn't know you were at risk."

"So *do* I have it?" Gabe asked. He had a moment of not wanting to know and then several moments when he thought of Christy who was young and didn't have the cloud of diabetes hanging over her. He heard the verdict with that thought in mind.

"Your fasting blood sugar is 124 mg%. We call that impaired glucose tolerance. I think we should call that diabetes. I'm going to order a glucose tolerance test for you this morning to see if you have it. You probably do, but it isn't a death sentence. If you begin treating the risk factors for heart disease that come with diabetes now, you don't have to be hurt by having diabetes. Usually it's heart and blood vessel disease that kills type 2 diabetics."

The doctor's words were meant to be reassuring, but Gabe couldn't be reassured. He spoke out of his gut reaction to the news.

"My mother was blind when she died," Gabe said. "She had kidney failure, and she died from a heart attack. I don't know that I believe the complications can be avoided."

"Come with me," the doctor said. "I want you to meet someone."

Gabe forgot about the time as he walked down the disinfected corridors. He was taken to a classroom. The doctor called the teacher from the room.

"This is Mr. Bodine. He's a diabetes educator here. Mr. Bodine, this is Mr. Killian. He has a high fasting blood sugar and may be diabetic. I consider Mr. Bodine an expert since he's had diabetes since he was thirty-nine. He's forty-seven now, and he doesn't have any damage from diabetes or blood vessel disease we can see. If you are motivated and compliant, Mr. Bodine can show you how to prevent the complications. That's why you wanted to be screened and why you want to start treatment now."

The educator shook Gabe's hand. "Come back when he's finished with you. I'll give you some basic education."

Gabe nodded like any number of dazed, newly diagnosed people and followed the doctor back to the exam room. He was given a lemon flavored bottle of glucose solution to drink and had blood drawn at one and two hours to assess his blood glucose response to the glucose load. He was shown a printout of his cholesterol, both good and bad, and his triglycerides. His triglycerides were 289 mg%. His total cholesterol was 220 mg%. They had never been high before.

"Your triglycerides are almost twice to top of the desirable range," the doctor said. "We need them to be under 150. Your cholesterol wouldn't look so bad if you didn't see the breakdown. Your good cholesterol or HDL is 29 mg%. It needs to be over 45. You want that number to be high so your body will move cholesterol out of your blood vessel walls. Your bad cholesterol or LDL needs to be under 100. Yours is 133 mg%.

"The reason why we have such a tight range is that we know people with type 2 diabetes have an 80 percent chance of dying from a heart attack. Even a newly diagnosed diabetic has the same risk of having a heart attack as someone who has already had a heart attack. It will usually happen within fifteen years of diagnosis. For that reason, I would recommend that you start on a cholesterol lowering medicine."

"Why can't I do something else with my diet?" Gabe asked. "I've read about those medicines. They can hurt your muscles and your liver. I'd rather not take that risk."

"That risk can be virtually eliminated when we monitor blood tests, Mr. Killian. The people that get into trouble with statin drugs usually have kidney disease or they are given another drug that makes the statin drug more toxic. Taking everyone we treat into consideration, your risk of even having an abnormal blood test is around five patients in a thousand. Your risk of heart disease is eight hundred out of a thousand. We know these medicines will cut your risk of heart disease from the first day you start taking them. They actually cut your risk of a heart attack even if your cholesterol is normal.

"It's your body and your choice, but if I develop any blood sugar elevation, I'll be taking one of them. The only thing you could do to lower your lipids on your own would be to increase your intake of fish oils like those that are in fatty fish like salmon and to lose more weight. You're within ten or fifteen pounds of ideal body weight now."

"Okay," Gabe said. "I understand." He felt trapped. It seemed reasonable to just agree to everything until he could walk away and think the situation through. He absorbed less than half of the information that was given to him. He listened to the doctor discussing the need for him to take aspirin because even people with glucose intolerance clot too easily. He was told his blood pressure was too high at 144/98. He was ready to insist to the doctor that the stress had caused it to go up. It was even higher when the doctor checked it.

"Young people at ideal body weight don't increase their blood pressures because of stress," the doctor said. "That's a characteristic of high blood pressure. You lose the ability to keep your pressure down when you're stressed. I'd like you to monitor your blood pressure only when you are stressed and try to keep that number in the normal range." Gabe knew his expression was blank, and the doctor continued to press his case.

"Think about how you look for a slow leak in your car's tire, Mr. Killian. You overinflate the tire and the increased air pressure finds the leak. Every time you increase your blood pressure, you are damaging the walls of your blood vessels."

"Everything you're saying is news to me," Gabe said. "I thought I knew about diabetes. Give me something to read. I can deal with anything I understand."

What he really wanted was time to think. He couldn't bear to hear anymore risks. He fled from the VA with two prescription bottles and a glucose meter. Mr. Bodine taught him how to use the glucose meter and told him to test his sugar two hours after eating. The target sugar after eating was 140 or less. In the bag with the other contraband was a stack of layperson booklets on diabetes. The appointment had taken four hours. The two-hour drive back to Cherokee gave him too long to think about how many people he had seen die from diabetes and its complications. It seemed like an insurmountable task to survive the disease when he had already failed to avoid it. At some point it occurred to him that it wasn't fair to condemn Christy to life with someone who might fall apart before her eyes. That thought made him feel sick, but he couldn't put the thought out of his mind.

Gabe barely made it to the college in time for his class. Then he was trapped by the faculty meeting until well after six o'clock. For the last thirty minutes of the meeting and the duration of the drive, he was frantic to see Christy. He felt as if she were the only medicine that could ease his tortured mind. He drove to Bryson City hoping she would still be there or that he would meet her on the road. He was feeling hopeless, cornered and doomed on the road back to Cherokee. He couldn't bring himself to go home alone so he drove to Jonah's study hall.

"Your name could become 'Thunder Face' if you don't smile soon," Jonah commented. "Where is Christy? She seems to bring out the best in you."

"Bryson City," Gabe responded sharply. "I couldn't get out of the faculty meeting soon enough to get her. She lives up one of the mountain roads where there aren't any lights or visible driveways. If there were, I'd be up there looking for her now." He hesitated. "Then I thought maybe I was being given a message. Maybe I shouldn't keep seeing her. Maybe I'm not supposed to have a family."

"I don't believe that, Gabe. You have always wanted your own family, and you have a real gift with children..."

"I'm starting to develop diabetes," Gabe interrupted. "I failed the screening test at the VA. I had forgotten about my appointment until yesterday morning, and now I almost wish I hadn't gone. When I say that, I want to kick myself because that's what my mother would have said. I'm not going to die like she did without trying to fight for my life, but I feel like it wouldn't be fair to Christy to keep seeing her. I don't feel like I can promise her much of a future now."

He expected Jonah would hesitate to answer. His uncle had lost friends and family members to diabetes. Jonah's eyes never left Gabe's face. "You have the answer in your own words. Your mother chose to die. That doesn't mean she didn't love you, Gabe. She lost my brother. Being in prison let her lose you. Her sentence would have kept her in prison for twenty years. She never made any effort to treat her diabetes, and she was already losing her sight and her kidney function when they paroled her.

"I know you have feared you would develop diabetes. Probably you've prayed not to develop it. I know you are afraid that you won't be able to control it because you couldn't prevent it. I also know that God doesn't test anyone unless they are strong enough to deal with the test as a challenge. Diabetes is killing our people partially because everyone believes it as an inevitable death sentence. Maybe someone who is strong enough to accept the challenge of living with it needs to show everyone else that it can be defeated. Our days are numbered only by God. I have always believed He has a greater purpose for you."

Gabe felt the peace of Jonah's words as if they had come from God. His uncle had never been wrong, and as always he had offered hope.

"I wouldn't not fight," he said. "I understand what you're saying about my mother. I guess I'll never understand why she didn't try when I asked her to try for me, but maybe it wouldn't have made any difference." He thought of Christy and looked to Jonah for a fair and unbiased decision.

"Do you think it would be fair to Christy if I keep seeing her?" Gabe asked. "I really want to see her, Jonah.

Last night I felt like she was the one. It seemed so clear. I guess I need her to be my soul mate right now. When did you know Reba was the one for you?"

"I'm not sure I should answer you," Jonah said slowly. "You have your father's lack of patience, and since he was my brother it's a trait we share." He scanned his nephew's face. "I knew after the first date, Gabriel. I knew she was the one God meant for me to marry. I was afraid I would be wrong so we dated for six months before we told each other what we both had known from the first night. I could feel it between us the first time she touched me. My eyes were drawn to her as if they had a will of their own. If you've been praying for God to let you know if Christy is the one for you, then don't be afraid to wait for God's answer."

"I'm afraid of making a mistake," Gabe said. "My mother thought she was doing the right thing for both of us when she married Pritchard. I'd rather die alone than make that kind of mistake. Since I met Christy, all of that has seemed insignificant. If not for the diabetes, I could have asked her to marry me tonight, and that's not because I want to sleep with her. How will I ever know what I should do when I feel so desperate? I'm just like my mother was when she made her mistake."

Jonah took Gabe's arm and propelled him into the next room. "Watch the class for me, Ethan," he said. He closed the door behind them. "I've wanted to wait for you to feel right about talking, Gabe, but we need to talk before you carry all the baggage of your past into this relationship. Your mother was seventeen when she married. She had a full scholarship to UNC, and she passed it by to go with Adam. She made your father very happy before he died, and I will always be grateful that he knew such happiness before his death. He was twenty when he died. Your mother was eighteen. You know what her family situation was. They were poverty stricken. She thought the two of you would be a burden on both families.

"She married Pritchard when she was nineteen. When he turned into a monster, she was isolated from anyone who might have helped her in an environment where dark-skinned people were still second rate citizens to some degree. She was so young when the terrible things started. You weren't the only one abused. Before she died, she told me he had threatened to kill both of you if she left. She had scars all over her from being beaten. She must have loved you enough to die for you or she wouldn't have ever picked up that gun.

"If we had had the money to hire a lawyer who cared, she wouldn't have gone to prison. Even putting together all the savings all of us had wasn't enough to retain a lawyer. She asked us to save that money for you." He put his hand on Gabe's shoulder. "It's very easy to think you understand the motives of another person, but you're only guessing. Raynelle was very young, and she grew away from God for a while after Adam died. Your situations are very different.

"Everything that happens works for the good of those who love God, Gabe. It might be that facing diabetes is meant to help you forgive your mother. Just now, I saw your face. You understand some of her feelings as you never did before. You've had so many reservations about trusting another person. You can't hold onto to those barriers if you want what Reba and I have. Christy is young, and she won't understand why you hesitate to be close to her. If you love her, you will have to open every part of your soul to her. If you can't do that, you can't make the wedding vow to God. We both know that's really what marriage is. It's a three-way partnership with a man, a woman, and their God."

"It's odd how you can believe you know where you're going," Gabe said. "Yesterday I told my church class that we might be better off if we just followed the cloud of God's presence through the wilderness and believe He'll show us where we need to go. Now I'll have to live my advice."

Jonah escorted Gabe to the door. "I've believed that for a long time now, Gabe. I do understand how you feel about making that journey alone. Every man has a moment when he realizes he is alone on the earth. Remember Adam asked God to give him a companion. Before I married Reba, my father told me about all the years when he walked alone. He said he never prayed as hard about anything as he did about the decision to marry my mother. You've been alone for a long time. For my sake, make sure you do your part to make a perfect union."

"I will," Gabe said slowly. "Thank you for listening."

Jonah watched as his nephew walked to his truck. In the quiet darkness of the church foyer, he said a long, fervent prayer for Gabe and Christy.

Gabe drove around for an hour, flirting with the idea of climbing the mountainside that night. He focused on Christy instead of the turmoil in his mind. He went home just before eleven and found sleep impossible. Long after midnight, he sat on his living room floor with his open Bible in his lap, not reading. Job came into the living room several hours later rubbing his eyes and squinting at the clock.

"Do you know it's three o'clock in the morning, Gabe?" He sat down on the floor and looked at his cousin with concern. "Have you thought you might be kind of jumping into this relationship? Maybe you need to take a couple of deep breaths and try to clear your head. I mean, I like her, Gabe, but you've known her three days."

"I know." Gabe shook his head. "I've been sitting here for three hours trying to clear my head. I don't think anyone but Christy can clear it. For the last couple of years, every day went like the one before it. Now I feel like almost everything in my life has changed in a matter of days. I go to bed thinking of her and get up glad to see the morning because I'll get to see her again. I've been sitting here and praying for direction. When I opened my Bible, look where I landed." He pointed to Psalm 30:5.

Job read the verse as if to himself. "'For his anger endureth but a moment; in his favor is life: weeping may endure for a night but joy cometh in the morning.'"

"How many times did your father read that verse to me? It must have been twenty." Gabe looked at Job. "I think it's a sign that morning is finally coming for me, Job. That's how she makes me feel."

Job looked at Gabe with empathy. "Be sure, Gabe. You're thinking about forever. Forever is a long time."

Tuesday morning, Christy's leg felt sore all the way to her hip joint, and it hurt even more when she tried to stand. She cut off the bandage and poured more peroxide over it. The redness was spreading up her leg in streaks. She thought of climbing back into bed, but she knew it was wrong to give up on everything. She said a prayer to have some sign that she had a future. When she had finished, she knew she needed to walk down to the emergency clinic in Bryson City. She made it out of the bus. After ten feet, she knew she felt as if she was going to pass out. She had to sit down on the path until the pain eased and then crawled back into the bus. She was shaking with a chill as she swallowed two more anti-inflammatory pills and crawled back into her sleeping bag to get warm. She intended to sleep until the pain was better, but she slept until the world was dark all around her. Then she was too sick to even try to get up.

Gabe's special topics class met once a week and ended at five o'clock. As the clock struck the hour, he hurried through the crowd of students around his desk.

He sprinted to his truck and drove through rush hour traffic to Deep Creek Campground. Bo, the convenience store owner, was stacking inner tubes with Joannie when Gabe arrived. He looked alarmed when Gabe came to meet him.

"Have you seen Christy?" he asked Gabe. "I was hoping she was with you."

"Not since Sunday," Gabe replied anxiously. "Why?"

"She cut her leg Sunday night, and I chewed her out good about not getting medical help. It was already getting infected yesterday. When she didn't come to work today I thought she probably went to the clinic in town, but I called there to see about paying her bill. Nobody has seen her."

"Do you know where she lives?" Gabe asked. "I've dropped her off at a dirt road on the river, but she didn't want me to drive up."

Bo pointed to his office and took Gabe inside before he answered. "I could get myself in trouble by telling you this, but I've been worried about Christy for a while. I think she may be in a lot of trouble. She came here last fall and worked until we closed down. Then she worked in Bryson City at three of the restaurants. She gave everybody a different name and a different social security number.

"I confronted her about it, and she told me she had seen a murder. She said she had been running for her life since last fall. I tried to get her to call the police and do that federal witness thing, but she was freaking scared out of her mind. I've been paying her cash to keep her safe. I don't know if Murray is her real name or not."

"She told me it was Fielding," Gabe said. He had a sinking sensation in his chest. He thought Christy had deliberately deceived him, but something told him he needed to confirm his gut reaction. "I'm going to look for her," he told Bo.

"If you want some help, give me five minutes to close, and I'll go with you."

Gabe changed into shorts and a tee shirt in the rest room and then waited for Bo outside the store. He couldn't keep from staring at the mountainside where Christy had said she lived. When Joannie had finished her stack, she came over to him and spoke bluntly.

"You hurt her as much as the leg did. She only stuck it out yesterday because she thought you would come. When you find her, you might want to apologize."

Gabe couldn't reply to her accusation because it reaffirmed his own worries. He had said he would see Christy Monday night and then missed the narrow window of opportunity.

"If I didn't care about her, I wouldn't be here now," he informed Joannie tersely. "After I apologize, I'm going to make sure the distance isn't an issue anymore." He walked back to the office leaving a stunned Joannie beside the inner tubes.

Sunset was at eight o'clock, and the rain started at seven. It was a southern summer deluge that washed down the mountainside in rivulets. Gabe and Bo had a hard time keeping their footing and found no signs of any driveways or paths as the wind rose and slapped their faces with wet foliage. Bo gave up at 8:30, but Gabe drove back to Bryson City and bought a lantern. In the darkness, despite being soaked to the skin, he used all his Seal skills to explore every inch of the dirt road until it became a path. He found and explored nine abandoned cars with no signs they had been disturbed for many years.

With each find he grew more discouraged and began to wonder if what he had felt for Christy was one sided. He wondered if she had left Bryson City fearing he knew too much about her. He even wondered if there were another man she did love or if she were still emotionally involved with whoever had broken her heart.

When paranoia began to overtake him, he stopped in the rain and prayed that finding her or not finding her would be a sign.

Fifteen minutes later, he had his answer. Seemingly by chance he saw the narrow trail curling into the kudzu jungle and followed it to the bus. He was sure it wouldn't be the right place. He couldn't imagine that a twenty-one-year-old girl could live in such a place, but as his lantern shed light on the path into the bus, he knew it had been freshly made. He knew the stain on the metal strut under the steps was blood. He held his breath as he climbed into Christy's sanctuary and found her unconscious and barely responsive, curled inside her sleeping bag. As he knelt beside her, he could almost feel the heat from her fever radiating off her body. He shook her gently. That touch told him she was dangerously sick.

"Christy. It's Gabe. We've got to get you to a hospital."

She groaned, but her eyes never opened as he unzipped the sleeping bag and used the lantern to examine her. It didn't take long to find the source of her fever. Her leg was swollen twice its size and streaked with red and purple. Gabe had enough cross training as a medic to know Christy was very sick and could die. He shouldered her weight easily and pulled the sleeping bag across her body to keep the rain off her. Almost as an afterthought he put her backpack on his other shoulder. The quarter mile walk down the mountainside was difficult because of the slippery mud and layers of foliage.

Gabe fumbled with the truck door for several minutes before he could unlock it. He eased Christy down on the seat and secured her with the seat belt as best he could. He drove exceeding all the speed limits until a sheriff's deputy stopped him. Then, he had an escort to the county hospital in Bryson City. Just after midnight, he registered the girl he really didn't know. That lack of knowledge didn't keep him from being panic stricken for her as he sat in the waiting room. At midnight, he called his aunt and uncle for emotional back up.

Christy was in the emergency room for two hours and then went to intensive care. It was well after 2 A.M. when the doctor came to talk to Gabe.

"You're Christine Murray's boyfriend?" the doctor asked. When Gabe nodded, he continued, "What can you tell me about her?"

"I'm Gabe Killian. I've only known her a week. We met at Deep Creek Campground. She works at a store there. We've been out twice, and I was supposed to meet her yesterday. I was late and couldn't find her. When I came tonight, the store owner said she had cut her leg Sunday night and refused to get treatment. I was worried about her and went up the road where she said she lived looking for her. I found out she was living in an abandoned school bus. Her employer thinks she's been hiding because she was witness to a murder."

"We should call the police then," the doctor said.

"Please don't," Gabe requested. "This was all second hand. When she's better, I'll ask her. How is she?"

"She's in septic shock from a Streptococcal infection in her leg. That means the infection is in her blood stream. It's unusual for an infection to spread so quickly in a healthy young woman so we looked a little further. She's very anemic and suffering from malnutrition. The iron in her blood is almost undetectable. She must have been losing blood chronically for a long time. She's very ill, Mr. Killian. I don't know if she'll be all right, but if she makes it through today, I'll feel much better about her chances.

"She could use a transfusion, but she has a rare blood type, AB-. I've sent to Asheville for two units, but I don't know what they have to spare."

"I have AB- blood," Gabe said. "Can I donate for her?"

"I'll make arrangements for that. It would be a big help. I'll be back this evening and let you know how she's doing."

Gabe reached out to catch the doctor's sleeve. "Can I sit with her? She's going to be really scared when she comes around."

"I wish I could let you, but we have a small intensive care unit, and we'd have chaos if families were allowed in there all the time. You can visit every three hours, and if she's doing well, she'll be out tomorrow." As the doctor left the room, Jonah put a reassuring hand on Gabe's arm.

"She'll be all right. You got her here in time. You need some time to clear your mind, Gabriel. Get some sleep and teach your class. Either Reba or I will stay here in case she needs something."

"I can't leave her, Jonah," Gabe said adamantly. "Even if I'm never anything but her friend, I'm her friend, and I won't be guilty of abandoning people who need me. I already have my lesson plan for today, and it's water sample collection and analysis. If you could give the list to Dr. Collins, he'll send the students out, and I'll catch them up on Friday. Tell them to meet me in lab four on Friday at 8 A.M."

"At least try to get some sleep until the visiting hours," Jonah replied as he conceded defeat.

CHAPTER 8

It was still three hours before he could visit Christy when Gabe had donated a unit of blood for her. He forced himself to go home where he showered, changed clothes, and collected his laptop and lesson planner. He picked up a cup of coffee at the all night coffee shop across from the hospital and took a seat in the ICU waiting room. While waiting, he sent an e-mail to his best friend, Tracy Tolliver, from his Navy days. Tracy had left the Seals after being injured and now worked in Naval intelligence. Gabe also sent a lengthy e-mail to his department chairman at the college explaining his whereabouts and how he intended to cover his classes. Then he submitted his field reports to the National Park Service. By the time he had finished, the volunteer in the waiting room was calling visiting hours.

He was relieved to see some of the color had returned to Christy's face, but he didn't expect her to open her eyes and speak to him.

"Gabe, you've got to get me out of here!" she said frantically. "They'll find me now. If they do, they'll kill me." Gabe put a reassuring hand on her arm.

"I guess Fielding is your real name," he said. "I registered you as Christine Murray. That's the name Bo gave me." Christy closed her eyes in relief.

"I'll tell you about everything. I promise I will."

"You don't have to tell me now, Christy."

"I want to tell you. I almost told you on Sunday. I was just scared you wouldn't want to see me again." She closed her eyes and two tears rolled down her cheeks.

Gabe wanted Christy to need him. He had never felt like he was needed. He had not gotten over his mother's rejection of his offer to care for her. It had been a gaping void in his heart since her death. He moved even closer to Christy's side and wiped her tears.

"I'm not going to leave you, Christy. I hadn't let myself be involved with a woman until I met you. I want to take care of you no matter what it takes. I'm in love with you."

"You can't love me, Gabe," she sobbed. "You don't know me. I want you to love me more than anything, but I can't do it to you. I can't let you know who I am."

"I already know, Christy. We're just alike. We're both looking in control on the surface, but we aren't. We're just praying to hang on. I just want you to know that I'm here for you. You aren't alone."

She looked at him with disbelief and then her tears fell freely. "I really need you, Gabe. I've been so alone. I thought I was going to die. I didn't think anyone would really care if I did die."

The nurse stepped into the curtained cubicle and warned, "You have about five more minutes." Gabe sat on the edge of the bed.

"I looked for you for about four hours in the rain before I found you, Christy. I prayed for it to be a sign if I found you or if I couldn't find you. I kept looking for you because I care about you. I hope you believe me." He wiped her tears again hoping to see some sign that she trusted him. The only emotions he could read were fear and confusion. "You're really anemic. The doctor said you don't have any iron stores in your body. He needs to know why."

"I used to be a blood donor," she said. "I have a rare blood type, and I gave almost every month. Iron makes my stomach sick so I didn't take it like I was supposed to." Her gaze wavered, and Gabe knew she had told him only some of the truth. He chose not to push her.

"I'll tell the doctor. He can probably give you some iron while you're here."

"I don't have any insurance and no way to pay, Gabe."

"The hospital applied for state aid for you. They know you're indigent. Don't worry, Christy. Just get well."

"Time's up," the nurse said firmly.

"I'll be back in three hours," Gabe vowed. He bent and whispered in her ear. "Don't forget your name is Christine Murray."

She was smiling as he walked away, and Gabe felt even more protective and responsible for her. He went back to the waiting room and sat down to check his e-mail. The answer from Tracy Tolliver floored him.

"Hey Windrunner, it's good to hear from you. We need to get together sometime. I ran the search you wanted. Are you sure you have the right name and birth date? According to vital statistics, Christianna Fielding died last year. If you have anything else, I'll rerun the search. Tracy."

Gabe replied, "More later." Then he closed his computer and left the hospital for the sheriff's office.

Gabe knew all the police force in Cherokee and half the county sheriff's deputies because they had used him to train their SWAT teams after he returned to Cherokee. He had continued to work with them on all their training exercises. He decided to go to the sheriff's office because he was owed some favors and knew they would keep his confidence. The corporal on duty was Buddy Wolfson, and he came out to greet Gabe.

"Hey, Gabe. What's up?"

"I need your help, Buddy. I have a friend who's in trouble. I haven't known her very long, so she hasn't told me everything, but I know it's bad trouble. She was a witness to something bad. It might be Mafia connected. I need what I'm going to tell you to be between the two of us, at least for now."

"You've got it." Buddy sat down and pointed to the chair across from him.

Gabe sat down slowly and tried to think of how he should begin. "She said she saw a murder and the ones that did it know she saw it. She says she had to run because they tried to kill her. I gave her name and birth date to a friend of mine in Naval Intelligence, and he said the government's records say she died last year. I want to take her name and birth date and run a background search."

Buddy hesitated and then shook his head. "I'm not sure you want to run an unencrypted search, Gabe. If she saw a Mafia killing, they may really be looking for her. They may have their computers ready to pick up on any mention of her name, birth date, or social security number."

"What about the search Tracy ran?" Gabe asked anxiously.

"If he went through Naval Intelligence, it was encrypted. I can't do that, but I have a friend in the FBI. Give me the information, and I'll see what I can get." He pushed a pad of paper across the desk and Gabe wrote down the name and birth date.

"You ought to get a gun permit, Gabe," Buddy warned. "If she's telling the truth, trouble has a way of being contagious."

"I've had a permit since I got out of the Navy, Buddy. I don't have a problem with carrying or using my gun," Gabe said defiantly. "After all, I've been trained to handle trouble." As he walked to his car, he felt more protective toward Christy Fielding than he had ever felt toward anyone. Personal risk was not a consideration.

The doctor accepted Christy's story about being a blood donor and infused her with Gabe's blood and a bag of intravenous iron solution. He also started her on multiple vitamin supplements. That evening, with her fever down to 101°F, she was moved to a regular room. Gabe was already at her bedside when the stretcher brought her.

When she was safely transferred, the nurse took her vital signs and left them alone. Christy was silent for a long time until Gabe picked up her hand.

"I had the feeling you were trying to hide under the kudzu."

"That was the idea." She held his hand tightly but did not look at him. "I was enrolled at an art college in Tennessee. It's called Tucker. I had a scholarship that paid everything. Every year they had a blood drive for this girl with leukemia. They wanted people with AB- to give so they tested everybody. There weren't that many of us, so I always gave blood. There was a nurse named Chuck who took the blood. He knew I hated needles so he let me breathe gas like the dentists use.

"One day when I was a junior, I went to give blood, and I woke up in this strange place. It was like a prison. They kept us there to give blood every week and gave us shots to make us make more blood. No one ever got away except sometimes somebody disappeared. I think I really knew they were being killed, but I didn't want to believe it. I had been there about six months when I was the one they were going to kill. They sent me to give blood again, but I was the only one there that day. Usually there were a bunch of people like cattle being milked. Chuck was there, and he gave me the gas, but then he woke me up and took me out of the compound. He had keys to get out. It was dark, and I thought we were safe until the shooting started. They shot him in the back just as we made it to his car. I drove, and he told me where his house was. Finally we got there, but there were already people there. Chuck kept telling me where to go until we reached the interstate. Then he got quiet. He was dead." She was silent for a long time.

"I never watched anybody die before, and he died to get me away. It happened last September, but it still comes back to me like it was yesterday. I've spent a lot of hours praying to know why I deserved to live. I couldn't stand to see anyone else be hurt for me. Especially someone I care about. So I had to warn you. You can't take the risk of being with me." Her voice broke.

Gabriel felt sick for her because he was absolutely sure she was telling him the truth as she believed it. Though her story sounded incredible, he knew she couldn't have imagined it. He knew she might still be in danger. Even when Buddy's warning rose in his memory, Gabe didn't care that he might be at risk by being with her.

"You were a victim, Christy. You didn't do anything to earn what happened to you. Sometimes bad things happen to good people, and that doesn't make them any less good. The man who helped you gave his life, but it sounds like he owed it to you and the other people he helped kill. Maybe he earned himself a place in the next life because he knew you. If being with you is a risk, for me it's worth taking. I understand how you feel because I saw someone sacrifice their life for mine when I was a kid. I didn't know why I was spared so I just keep trying to return the favor."

"I couldn't watch it happen again," she said. "You're the only real friend I have now, but I can't let you get hurt because of me. I just need to go, Gabe. I just need to move to another place and keep running until they forget to chase me."

"Please don't go," he said. He kept his voice controlled, but he was feeling very desperate. "I couldn't run far enough to forget how you make me feel. I hope you won't run when I ask you to stay." He moved to sit on the edge of the bed and held both of her hands. He spoke impulsively out of his fear of losing her.

"I can keep you safe if you'll let me. Just come home with me. I'll make sure Job is always there at night so no one will think anything is going on. I doubt they'd expect to find you on the Cherokee reservation. For that matter, we could get married. It doesn't have to be physical if you aren't sure of how you feel. I just want to be able to protect you without leaving us open to gossip. I've made a big deal at church talking to the kids about not having premarital sex. I don't want them to think I'm a hypocrite. When this is over, you can have the marriage annulled if you don't want to stay married."

Christy had felt like someone's duty for too many years after her grandmother's death. She couldn't see that the way Gabe had asked her was driven by his own insecurity. She felt as if her situation would doom their relationship. Even when she wanted to accept him, she spoke carefully and tried to put some distance between them.

"I always thought when someone asked me to marry them, it would be moonlight and roses instead of hospitals and desperation. I don't want to be alone in this anymore. I don't think it's fair to you, but I'm glad you're willing to help me."

Gabe regretted making his offer sound as if it were just for convenience. He knew he was using her desperation as an excuse. The offer seemed his best chance to assure their continued relationship. His main concern was that her answer hadn't been a clear acceptance. That thought reopened his scars of poor self esteem, the inevitable legacy of childhood abuse. The nurse came to administer an antibiotic and a pain pill before they could talk more. The latter made Christy sleep. Gabe sat beside her until exhaustion claimed him for the night.

The doctor's arrival awakened both of them early the next morning. He greeted them and then moved to examine Christy's leg. The redness was receding rapidly, and the swelling was all but gone.

"It looks really good, Miss Murray. I'm going to change you to an oral antibiotic tonight. If you're doing this well tomorrow, I'll let you get out of here if you promise to give up your previous quarters."

"I promise," Christy said without any signs of happiness. Gabe saw her reaction as a sign of her reservations. He had a hard time concealing his disappointment even when he knew his expectations were probably unrealistic.

"I'll make sure she's all right," Gabe vowed. "My aunt will be sitting with her today. I teach at the college, and I have two classes I can't miss."

"Will you be gone long?" Christy's pleading panic-stricken expression made Gabe feel more secure in her feelings for him.

"I'll only be gone five hours." He looked at the doctor. "Is there any chance she could go home with me tonight? I guarantee she'll do whatever you say."

"I'll check her again this afternoon," the doctor conceded, "but she's lucky to be progressing this fast."

When the door closed behind the doctor, Christy sat up and reached for Gabe's hand. "I'm scared, Gabe. I don't feel safe here. I don't think my leg is as much of a danger as what I told you."

"They don't know you're here, Christy. Before they have time to find you, we'll have you checked out of here and staying at my house. I promise I won't be gone very long."

"Don't leave until Reba comes," she begged. "Please."

"I won't, Christy. Just trust me. I'll be here for you for the rest of your life if you want me to be."

She reached out to him like a child, and he held her in his arms, feeling the need to protect her growing even stronger. He also felt a transmission of her fear and left her reluctantly even when Reba was installed beside her bed.

CHAPTER 9

Christy found Reba to be a soothing presence, and she made an effort to relax and talk about Gabe. The more Reba told her, the more Christy had to realize that she was seeing only what Gabe had allowed her to see.

Reba was obviously very proud of Gabe and thought of him as her son. She told Christy more about the injury that had ended his Navy career. Christy didn't understand that Reba was really trying to give her more insight into how selfless Gabe was.

"We'll never know where it happened. Everything the Seals do is classified even when it's over, and there are some teams that are more classified than others. Gabe was on an anti-terrorism team. They went on the most dangerous missions. They drop the Seal teams off at sea to swim to shore usually at night and then come back to get them. When Gabe's team returned to the shore, they were ambushed before they could get in the water. They were running across the docks trying to reach the water when the team leader was shot. Gabe was the only other officer, and he went back for him. He shot some of the men who were after them. He was shot in the shoulder, and the impact of the bullet made him fall off the dock. He fractured his skull, several ribs and his left leg. We didn't even know he was hurt for two weeks. Since the Seals operate covertly, he was flown to an aircraft carrier just after it happened. They flew him to Florida for surgery, and he was on a ventilator in a coma for a week. The doctors at Virginia Beach told us the coma was medically induced to keep his brain from swelling. They said that and the fact that they made his body very cold is why he has so little permanent impairment. They contacted us when they brought him back to Virginia Beach to recover.

"I think recovering at Virginia Beach was the worst part for Gabe. He had always tried to avoid being stationed there because of all that happened in Virginia Beach when he was a little boy. His Seal team operated out of Virginia Beach, but he wasn't ever on the base very long until he was hurt.

"He was terribly sick at first. He couldn't see, and he couldn't walk. He had been there for six weeks when they told him the peripheral vision loss would be permanent. He had a hard time coming to terms with it. He wanted to think it would come back eventually. The Navy gave him a Silver Star, and he was promoted to lieutenant commander. They would have transferred him to another job, but Gabe loved being a Seal. He didn't want to be in the Navy if he couldn't be in special forces.

"When they said he would have to be transferred, he took a medical discharge and let us bring him home. It was very difficult for him to make the transition. His mother was very ill by then, and it was several months before he had physically recovered from his injuries. I don't think he felt at home here until he finished graduate school and began defending his dissertation. That was when his mother died." Reba searched Christy's face.

"He's very serious about you, Christy. Maybe you think he's just your friend, but he wants more than that.

If you aren't very serious about him, please don't let him think you are. I've loved Gabe as if he were my flesh and blood since he was six years old. Jonah and I had been trying to have a baby for a year when the call came asking us to take Gabe. I thought he was the answer to my prayer, and I still believe he was. He was also a lesson that blessings take work. It was over a year before he accepted us and probably four years before he felt he was our son. Then we lost him when his mother came home. That was almost as hard as when I thought he might die." She looked at Christy with anguish in her eyes.

"If he reaches out to you and you push him away, he'll be terribly hurt. He might not ever get over that hurt because it has taken him twenty-five years to reach out to someone. If you just want his help or you don't know what you want, keep some distance between the two of you."

"What happened to him, Reba?" Christy asked. Gabe had seemed like a tower of strength to her, and she knew Reba was telling her that was exactly the image he intended to project. Reba hesitated as she weighed her alternatives. She was convinced that Christy was very fond of Gabe, and she knew Gabe was very emotionally involved with her. Reba made the maternal decision to try and push Christy to decide if she wanted Gabe sooner rather than later.

"I would prefer if this were between us, Christy. I'm not sure Gabe would want me to tell you, but I've prayed about it, and I think you need to know. His mother remarried after his father was killed. The man was also in the Navy, and Raynelle met him on the base. She wanted Gabe to have a father, and I don't think she took enough time to know Pritchard. After they married, it was obvious he didn't want to raise another man's son. He was very abusive to Gabe and Raynelle. I don't understand how someone could deliberately hurt such a young child, but Pritchard beat both of them frequently from the time

Gabe was two until he was six. He would start with beating Gabe and then beat Raynelle when she tried to protect Gabe. I'll never understand why she didn't just leave him. She had a home here, but I think she felt she would dishonor her family if she divorced. We didn't know about the abuse until it was too late. I can't bear to think of what Gabe went through.

"One night, Pritchard was beating Gabe, and Raynelle said she knew he was going to kill her baby. She shot her husband with his handgun. She was so angry and scared that she kept shooting him until he was dead. The police called it manslaughter, and she went to prison for ten years. People didn't listen to testimony about abuse then. Gabe had nine healed fractures from being beaten, and those are just what you can see.

"If he didn't have a strong spirit, his childhood would have destroyed him. We went with him to counseling for years. Children who are abused develop deep- seated problems with self esteem and trust. We tried to keep him safe and heal his heart, but his relationship with his mother thwarted that to some degree.

"Gabe felt like his mother sacrificed herself for him, and he wrote to her constantly when she first went to prison. Raynelle felt like he would be better off without the stigma of a mother in prison so she wouldn't see him. She never even answered his letters. He was sixteen when she came home, and Gabe didn't have a relationship with her. He had lived with us most of his life, but he thought it was his duty to care for his mother. She kept pushing him away until he was almost too angry and depressed to function. When he decided to join the Navy at seventeen, we agonized about it. Jonah was his guardian, and after we had prayed about the decision, he signed permission for Gabe to go. It was a good decision. Away from home, he learned to believe in himself.

"His mother realized what she had done after he left home, but it was too late to repair the damage between them. They never learned to communicate even when Gabe came home. I think that's why he hasn't let himself get involved with anyone before you. I think he's gotten past his trust issues because he thinks you need him."

Christy shuddered as Gabe's words echoed in her head. "I saw someone give up their life for me." The words told her that he did understand how she felt about Chuck's death. She thought he had lived through so many years of risking his life that he really didn't see her situation as threatening. It was obvious that he understood what sort of danger he might face. She let herself think that accepting his offer might not be wrong.

"I really care about him, Reba," Christy said. "How I feel is not because I need his help. When he's gone, all I can do is think about him. When I close my eyes, I see his face like I've known him all my life. I'm an orphan and after my grandma died, I didn't want to be close to anyone again because of how bad it hurt to lose them. When I'm with Gabe, that doesn't matter. I couldn't ever take advantage of him."

"It sounds like you're in love." Reba said. "I still remember the first time I felt that way about Jonah. It was the day we met, and that feeling hasn't ever gone away. Just be certain, Christy. I believe God only makes one man for every woman. If people don't wait to find that person, they destroy at least two lives."

Buddy came to the college to see Gabe just as he was leaving that afternoon. He had an envelope and a grim expression. "Your friend was reported missing from Tucker Art College in September of 1998 and then her records at Vital Statistics were deleted as if she's dead, but there isn't any death certificate. My contact at the FBI thinks someone hacked into the system and made her dead. I told them to let it ride like that. They're coming to interview her. Apparently other people have disappeared from that college, but they never had any leads until now." His face was anxious. "Gabe, I was ready to tell you to blow it off, but this smells like an organized crime thing. Those people don't see time as a barrier, and there's no statute of limitations on murder. You should really just turn her and this whole business over to the FBI as soon as you can."

"Everything worth doing and having has some risk, Buddy."

"This is different, Gabe. You had a license to kill when you were in the service. You can't fire on anybody now unless they fire on you first, and you'd better be able to prove it. Just saying you're threatened isn't enough. Look at what happens to us in law enforcement. I can shoot the biggest scum bag in North Carolina while he's chasing me with an ax and have his family sue me the next day for hurting poor innocent Bubba."

"I hear you, Buddy," Gabe said. His answer was designed to reassure his friend. "I would tend to be too quick on the trigger. Thanks for chilling me out."

When they parted, Gabe hurried to his truck realizing that he wanted to see Christy as if it were a physical need. The distance to the county hospital seemed almost insurmountable in the afternoon traffic. Than he was trapped behind a wreck for an hour. The only thing to occupy him during the wait was the stack of diabetes education materials. Gabe read them out of desperation. They weren't reassuring. They talked about all the possible complications and how excellent sugar control, cholesterol control and blood pressure control was necessary to prevent them. He still wondered if preventing them was really possible. He stuck his finger for the first time while sitting in the traffic jam. During the twenty second count, he told himself the reading would be a sign. He had eaten an hour earlier. The reading was 134.

"Okay," he prayed. "I'll believe I can do this, but I don't want to do it alone unless that's the way You want me to do it. Show me what to do about Christy." As he opened his eyes, the wall of cars began moving. He was at the hospital ten minutes later and took the stairs two at a time. The doctor had already arrived and was examining Christy's leg.

"I guess I'll have to eat my words," he admitted. "Your immune system is taking care of the problem, and your white blood count is down to normal. You can go home with Mr. Killian, but I need to see you in clinic on Monday. I want you back here immediately if your leg starts looking worse." He wrote out a prescription and put it on the bedside table. "That's for the antibiotic. Do you think you'll need anything for pain?"

"I hate feeling drugged," Christy said. "I'd rather hurt." Gabe smiled because they shared the same sentiment on that point, too.

"Thank you for everything, Doctor," Gabe said.

"You're welcome. You did a good job finding her and getting her here." The doctor bade them farewell and left to finish his rounds.

"Let's get out of here," Christy said in relief.

"Sounds good to me. I had my fill of hospitals when I was hurt." Gabe looked at his aunt. "Thanks, Reba. You've been great as always." He saw his aunt to the door and then closed it before returning to sit beside Christy. "The bad news is you don't have any clothes to wear. I brought your backpack down the mountainside, but it got soaked with mud and rain. I'll go across the street to the discount store. I can fill your prescription there and pick up some clothes for you. What size do you wear?"

"It was eight, but I think I've lost some weight. Just get the jogging stuff. It's stretchy." She moved suddenly as if compelled to move and slipped into his arms. "I really missed you. I've never felt that way about anyone but my grandmother. It's worse than being hungry."

He closed his arms around her protectively. Protectiveness rapidly accelerated into desire. They were locked together when the nurse entered the room.

"You might want to save the homecoming for when you get home," the nurse said. Even Gabe blushed, but Christy's fair skin made her embarrassment obvious.

"I'll shower while you shop," she said to Gabe.

"I'll be right back." He left her very reluctantly. The embrace and her welcome had rekindled his need to make her his own. As he roamed the aisles of the discount store, he decided to ask her to marry him without making excuses as to why. He knew people who had met and married after a matter of days and lived happily together. He was certain they could have that outcome if they put their reservations aside. It felt very right to shop for her and not awkward even when he bought her a package of plain cotton underwear. Dressing her made him feel as if she were his wife already.

He returned to the hospital with enough clothes for a weekend trip. The one possible snag hit him as he walked into the hospital with clothes she could wear out.

"Christy, do you have any ID?" he asked her. She was sitting on the bed in a clean hospital gown with her long red hair damp on her shoulders. She looked momentarily panic stricken.

"I hope so. Chuck was able to get my driver's license and birth certificate before we escaped. They're in my wallet in the front pocket of my backpack." Gabe put the sack of clothes on the bed and bent to examine the pack.

"It's still here," he reassured her. He handed her the wallet, and she thumbed through a wad of damp one dollar bills to extract her driver's license. It was a photo ID.

"Why?" she asked.

"You can't get married without a valid ID." He scanned her face for her response. She still hadn't come to a clear decision about what to do and hesitated to answer. It was physically painful for Gabe when she didn't respond in any way. Like anyone who has been rejected and abused, Gabe began putting up barriers to protect himself.

"You can't even get a library card without photo ID these days. I'll wait outside while you get dressed." He left the room before she could think of what to do or say.

In the hospital corridor, Gabe leaned against the wall and agonized that Christy didn't share his intense feelings. He wondered if she only wanted to be with him for protection and cared enough that she didn't want to lie to him. The latter worry cast a shadow over his relief because she had recovered. The buried worries about his health and long-term battle against diabetes came back to overwhelm him. He had slept very little over the previous two days, and he closed his eyes.

"Okay," he thought. "I'm not praying enough. I'll try to have patience and pray." He was praying when Christy touched his shoulder.

"Are you all right?" she asked with concern.

"Just tired," he said. "I almost fell asleep on guard duty. Are you ready to go?"

"Absolutely. I'm still limping a little, but it doesn't hurt like it did on Monday." She limped back to the bed and extended the money from her wallet to him. She meant it as a gesture to put them on more equal footing. That wasn't how Gabe took it.

"I know this isn't half of what you spent..." she began.

"I don't want your money, Christy," he interrupted. He felt as if she had slapped his face. "I have enough money to help out a friend in need." He lifted her muddy pack and walked back to the door. "I'll tell the nurse you're ready to leave."

Gabe had a hard time hiding his response to Christy's actions. He saw it as a clear attempt to keep distance between them. It was something his mother would have done and had done more than once. It told him that Christy either didn't care to read his feelings or just didn't care for him. He had to put himself into Seal mode to suppress his feelings. He told himself that she was simply a duty until the agony of rejection eased. He was in control at least on the surface when he returned. He told himself he was ready to protect her without expecting anything in return.

The nurse wheeled Christy to the door while he drove his truck to meet them. He hid all the diabetes materials under the seat. When she was seated inside, he closed the truck door and climbed into the driver's seat without a word. The silence was not comfortable as they drove down the expressway. They returned to Cherokee without any words being said. The silence became frightening for Christy. She had lived from moment to moment for a long time. It seemed almost impossible to think of having a future. When she realized she might have lost the chance to be with Gabe, she knew she was more afraid of that than being killed.

"I hurt your feelings," she said desperately. "I didn't mean to. I'm sorry, Gabriel." She put her hand over his hand gently. "I've felt helpless for months now. You're so certain of what to do. I just wish I could feel that way."

"I'm not sure I know what to do, Christy, which means it wasn't fair for me to ask you what I asked. I haven't had this kind of relationship before now. It's always been a superficial thing for me to date. I feel like you have control over every thought I have, but I know that feeling has to go both ways to make a relationship last. I want forever. I don't believe anything other than forever is right." He forced a grim smile. "We've had some terrific time together, but we were only showing our good sides. Now we're seeing all of our insecurities and bad traits. We both obviously have major trust issues. I'm a control freak. If I weren't sleep deprived, I probably wouldn't have taken all this so personally. Tomorrow, we'll start over. I've never been one to make snap decisions, but when I make up my mind, I don't usually change my mind. That's a Windrunner trait."

"Windrunner?"

"My middle name. It was my mother's family name and my nickname in the Navy. A long time ago, a man might have the name his parents gave him as a boy and then take another name when he was a warrior. That name would be descriptive. My great great great grandfather was named Windrunner. He was a messenger and ran between villages carrying the news. Since smoke signals and drum beats couldn't be used in these mountains, the runners were very important people.

"After the people were conquered, we had to have family names to live in a white world. Windrunner's name became his family's last name. Seal team members have a code name so I took the name Windrunner. Gabriel was my paternal grandfather's name. When I was a kid, he was still alive so I was Gabe since he was Gabriel."

"Gabriel fits you," she said timidly. "You look like the angel Gabriel to me. Do you want me to call you Gabe instead?"

"No. I actually like the way it sounds when you say my name. I can't say I feel like anybody's angel. I've never felt like I've earned my grandfather's name. He was everything I want to be." She thought he would say more, but he just kept driving while she struggled to make conversation. Gabe's thoughts drifted out of the truck to his grandfather. That Gabriel Killian had seemed fearless, but Gabe could remember his grandfather's definition of courage.

"Real courage is facing your greatest fear and knowing God will give you a strong heart to defeat it," he had said. The words seemed prophetic at that moment. Gabe's greatest fear had been a lifetime of being alone. He was certain he feared that more than diabetes. He thought he had moved more quickly in his relationship with Christy than he should have for that reason. It was obvious that Christy wasn't overwhelmed by the need to be with him even though she needed protection. He thought Christy's uncertainty was a message from God that they weren't meant to be together. He refocused on her voice with difficulty.

"Christianna was my Swedish grandmother's name. My middle name is Claire. That was my mom's name. That's all I have of her now. I had pictures and keepsakes, but I guess they destroyed all of them when they took me to the compound." She turned to stare at his face, feeling the pull to touch him even then. He ignored her gaze even when it caused a palpable warmth on his cheek.

"I do trust you," she said. "I never felt this way before either, Gabriel. I can't stop thinking about you. I don't want to stop thinking about you." The words made Gabe feel less rejected, and he turned his hand under hers so their fingers could entwine. He regretted the concession almost immediately. Touching her made him feel as if there were hope of having her. After a few moments, he put both hands on the wheel and kept his eyes on the road. He had charted his course away from hers. Turning back would only bring more pain.

"We'll just use this time to get to know each other better." He pulled into the driveway and cut the ignition. "Let's get some supper, and then I'm going to get some sleep."

CHAPTER 10

Gabe had a headache before Job arrived. Job was a born entertainer and knew Christy was important to his cousin so he talked nonstop from the moment he came home. The noise and the lingering stress finally sent Gabe to the medicine cabinet though he rarely took medicine. As he held the bottle of pain medication in his hand, he wondered if he had even more reasons to have a headache. He went to his bedroom, locked the door and found his mother's blood pressure cuff. When he checked his blood pressure, it was 160/99.

He thought of the previous six months and realized he had had headaches more frequently than usual. They had all been associated with stress, and they were identical to the band-like headache he was having that night. He wanted to lay all the blame on stress, but he knew he had been in very stressful situations as a Seal and had never had any blood pressure elevation. He had to accept that the number in the clinic might be his average.

It was like another sign that he was already damaged by diabetes. The memories of his mother's death had never seemed more vivid. He told himself it wouldn't be fair to inflict that burden on a potential spouse. He also knew he owed the people who knew him the courage of fighting diabetes even if he chose to be alone with his battle. That was his only incentive when he decided to take the medication he had been given. He consoled himself with the thought that keeping his blood pressure under 130/80 was his most powerful weapon in cutting his risk of heart and kidney disease.

He left his jacket in the bedroom and returned to the truck to collect the two prescription bottles and the other materials from the VA. Christy was in the kitchen and didn't come out to question his actions. He took the paper bag to his room and took the blood pressure pill along with an aspirin. The cholesterol medication and the blood pressure medication were labeled to take in the morning. He decided taking the blood pressure medication then and the next morning wouldn't hurt him when his blood pressure was so high.

He had no desire to eat and ignored the meal Christy had prepared. He put his gun on the stereo and donned his headphones. He stretched out on the floor beside the stereo and medicated himself with music.

"Lock up, Job," he said. "I'm not much of a watchman right now."

Christy felt rejected by his actions, but she knew the distance between them was of her own making. She sat down on the floor beside the bookcase to look at the photo albums Reba had compiled for Gabe. Job sat beside her and told her who the people were.

"Gabe looks like his dad," Christy told Job. "And sort of like your dad. Of course, he didn't even look like himself when he didn't have hair." The pictures fascinated her. She had been seeing Gabriel as a man and not as a Native American man. As she looked at the record of his past life, she realized how many things he had told her testified to how strongly he was committed to his ethnic roots. She had never been close friends with a person of another race. It made knowing Gabe and his family seem even more special.

"He was almost eighteen when he enlisted," Job said. "His hair was really long then, but he got shaved just like every other recruit." He flipped back two pages and showed her the picture of Gabe's high school graduation. His dark hair was tied back, and his expression made Christy smile.

"His rebel without a cause phase."

"Oh, he had causes," Job said. "He had all sorts of causes. Gabe puts his heart into everything he does." He turned forward to a photograph of Gabe in fatigues. "This picture was taken the day he graduated from basic training. He did so well on the aptitude test that he got to go to the warrant officer's school after his first tour. He was accepted to the Seal training program when he was twenty." Job turned the page and pointed to a picture of Gabe in camouflage. "That was taken when he finished the Seal training in San Diego. I think he lost thirty pounds in six months. We almost didn't recognize him when he came home on leave. That's when he qualified as a parachutist." Job grinned.

"He was absolutely freaking fearless. He was awarded six medals while he was a Seal." He flipped the page and indicated Gabe in a cap and gown. "He graduated from college and went to officer's candidate school when he was twenty-four. That's one of the times he was assigned to submarine duty. This is where he graduated from OCS and made lieutenant." He flipped the pages and showed her the pictures of Gabe in his dress whites. Christy smiled because Gabe looked so very handsome with his dark skin against the white uniform.

"He looks good in his uniform."

"He's a warrior," Job said intently. "To be a warrior means so much more than just a word. I wanted to follow in his footsteps, but when he almost died, it freaked my mother out. He'd been hurt before, but the last time was really bad. My mother and my sister started giving me a hard time about going to college here. Then, Gabe, the traitor, took their side so here I am."

"In college and loving it," Christy surmised. "Gabe seems to like having you here."

"He'd rather have *you* here. Gabe really likes you, Christy," Job said. "How do you feel about him?" Christy flushed as she looked at Job.

"You're very nosy, Job Killian."

"Gabe is more than family to me," Job asserted. "He's been my best friend since he came home from the Navy. He's not a person you can get to know very easily, but I know him. Most people couldn't have come through what he's been facing since he was real young. He doesn't deserve to be hurt again. If you don't feel the way he does, don't string him along."

Christy looked at Gabe's sleeping form without answering Job. For the first time, she realized he was as emotionally vulnerable as she was. His offer to marry her replayed itself in her mind until she knew it wasn't an offer to protect her. She knew Gabe had been offering himself to her body and soul. Those thoughts were still circling in her mind when Job went to the kitchen to clean up. She heard him turn off the lights and lock the back door. A few minutes later, she heard his bedroom door close.

Then, she felt very alone and moved to lie down beside Gabe. Even that closeness wasn't enough. She had felt alone and isolated for years. She wanted and needed the closeness that they had between them lying in his back yard. Hesitantly, she reached out and rested her hand on his arm. Gabe sat up almost immediately and put the headphones on the stereo case. The movement dislodged her hand. Christy knew it was deliberate.

"What time is it?" He glanced at the clock on the wall. "I never thought I'd sleep this long." He looked at Christy as if she were simply a guest in his house.

"You shouldn't be sleeping on the floor when you just got out of the hospital. Sleep in my room. I'll sleep on the couch."

"I'm not really tired." She reached out to put her hand on his arm again and spoke pleadingly. "Could we talk for a little while? I'll make you some hot tea."

"That sounds good." Gabe stood and offered her his hand, which she didn't hesitate to take. He released it as soon as she was on her feet. He didn't want his physical response to Christy to give him hope again.

"How's your leg feeling?" he asked as if she were an acquaintance.

"It's not bad." She went to the tea canister and took two cups out of the cabinet. "Do you want me to fix something for you to eat?"

"I'm not really hungry." Gabe sat down at the table and watched Christy make the tea. He felt the same emotional response he had felt when she had cooked for him, but his self defenses killed the thought. He thought Christy was probably still trying to repay him. The thought made him want to leave the kitchen. The silence was heavy between them.

"You don't owe me anything, Christy," he said. "I offered to help you, and I don't want to be repaid. Even if we're just friends, I wouldn't expect anything in return for helping you. I think I probably shouldn't have tried to make our relationship more for just that reason. I wouldn't have wanted to you to marry me because you owed me something. I felt like we were on the same wavelength. The truth is we don't know each other, and we don't have that much in common. I haven't let myself get close to many people so my relationship skills aren't good. I obviously put you on the spot. I won't do it again."

Christy knew he was ending their closeness with his words. She turned with fear on her face. At that moment, she felt as if she had let the last three years of her life make her incapable of responding without fear and paranoia.

"It isn't like that," she said. "I really feel connected to you. I've never felt so connected to anyone. That couldn't be by chance. I just know I've been a burden for you. I've dreaded living that way since my grandmother died."

Her words made Gabe angry at that moment. He felt as if she were stringing along his battered emotions.

"You seem so fearless," she said. "And certain about how you want your life to be."

"Only a fool is fearless," he snapped. "I don't relish the idea of being alone for the rest of my life, but I want to marry my soul mate. I lived in the middle of a very unhappy marriage, and I'd rather be alone than live that way again. That's one of the things that haunts me. I try not to think of those things. That doesn't mean they aren't in the back of my mind. Today I was worrying about our relationship, and I prayed for God to show me the right path. I don't believe anything happens without a reason. It's obvious you have a lot of reservations about any long-term commitment to me. When you showed me how you felt, that was my answer. I read more into what you were wanting than I should have. You won't hurt me if you tell me that you just want my help."

"No," she said frantically. "That wasn't what I was saying."

"Then please tell me what you want," he said in frustration. "I'm the kind of person who lives by what my objective is. I need to know where you want to go."

"I want to go with you," she said. "I want to be with you. I just wanted to feel like I could give you something. I don't want to wake up married to someone who wishes they hadn't asked me. I don't have anything, Gabriel. I don't know why you would want me."

It seemed very simple in that moment. Gabe couldn't see that Christy was in love and terrified for him. He decided that neither of them was capable of trusting the other. His expectations of love couldn't rationalize her behavior, and he felt too fragile to risk further rejection. He gave up, but he didn't have it in him to be vengeful. His agenda changed to not hurting Christy while protecting himself.

"Let's just put today behind us, Christy. You're safe with me. Stay here for a few days and decide what you want to do. This isn't a spur of the moment decision no matter what the circumstances seem to be."

She put her arms around him and held him tightly. He put his arms around her but more as a gesture of comfort. She pressed her face against his neck and clung to him. She wanted to feel that he wanted her. She felt no response. He pushed her back gently and walked her to his bedroom door.

"The sheets are clean. I haven't been home to sleep since I changed them."

"Could you lay down and just hold me?" she begged. "We could leave the door open."

"I can't," he said. He hoped she didn't know that he wanted to hold her. "That's too close for both of us right now. Get some sleep."

He walked away before she did and returned to lay down on the couch. He couldn't think about anything except the possibility of life with Christy. It was hard to close his mind to the thought. He slept only intermittently.

CHAPTER 11

Gabriel awakened when he heard Job emerging from his room. He could almost feel the grim expression on his face. He felt as if a part of him had died. His cousin looked into the living room with concern.

"Are you feeling better?"

"Yeah," Gabe said. "I'm making it. God's still trying to teach me that His ways aren't always what I want." He sat up and rubbed his eyes. The headache was gone though his tension was no less. "I think I'll get a shower. Would you put on some hot water for tea?"

"No problem." Job hesitated as if he wanted to say more and then went into the kitchen. Gabe took his workout bag to the bathroom because his other clothes were in the bedroom with Christy. He showered and changed clothes knowing he would have to dress for class when he had access to his closet.

In his room, Christy had awakened and was digging through the various shopping bags to find the new clothes Gabriel had bought her. She found the sack of diabetes materials quite by accident. She flipped through them thinking Gabe had them because of his mother.

When she found the two bottles of medication in the bag and saw they were dated the day he had missed their appointed meeting, she knew the books were his. It occurred to her that Gabe might not have made it to the campground on Monday for a very different reason than the one she had surmised. She replaced them in the bag and left it exactly as she had found it. She didn't feel she had the right to ask him about the medicine or Monday. She was praying he would be open to her again.

When she heard Gabe leave the bathroom, she went to the shower. She spent thirty minutes trying to make herself look pretty and desirable. Since her only clean clothes were the new jogging suits, she couldn't meet her objective.

Gabe went into his room and dressed for his class. He took the two pills and an aspirin. He put the sack in his dresser drawer and tucked the testing kit into his jacket pocket. He put on his handgun and took his blood pressure as an afterthought. Despite the lingering stress of the previous hours, his blood pressure was 126/72. He couldn't feel any side effects from having taken the medicine. He was wondering if taking blood pressure medicine would do anything to him that he couldn't foresee. He had heard a certain number of horror stories about sexual problems in men on blood pressure medicine. He put the thought out of his mind. He hadn't slept with anyone in thirteen years and didn't intend to until he was married. That seemed unlikely. It was the kind of issue his mother would have worried over. It was an excuse to not follow the doctor's advice.

Job was eating a scrambled egg and gestured toward a full mug of tea. "I fixed extra eggs," he said.

"I'm still not hungry." Gabe sat down with the mug cradled in his palms. "I'll probably be home late. I need to go to Asheville again. I'll either take Christy with me or leave her at your parents' house."

"Asheville?" Job echoed. "The VA?"

"Yeah," Gabe said. "Do yourself a favor and give up all the sugar and fat now. You won't like the payback." Job's eyes were eloquent, but he read Gabe's expression and didn't ask. He didn't have to ask to know Gabe was facing several major challenges at once.

"If you need anything, just ask," Job said. "I'll always be here for you, Gabe."

"I know," Gabe said. "It's all right. Remember, God never gives you more than you can stand." He stood as Christy entered the kitchen. "I'm going to walk for a half hour. I need to leave at 8 o'clock. Can you be ready?"

"I'm ready now," she said.

"Get something to eat first," Gabe said. "I do lunch late on Friday." He left the house and started walking toward the river. Before he was halfway down the driveway, Job had confronted Christy.

"Just leave," Job said as he left the table. "You're not being fair to Gabe. He has enough to worry about without worrying about your problems when you obviously don't care about his."

"Is he mad at me?" Christy asked like a frightened child.

"He's hurting, and I think we both know why." Job put his dishes in the sink and left the kitchen. He slammed the door to his bedroom. He was shocked when Christy knocked. He snatched the door open and glared at her.

"You just don't get it, do you?"

"I love him," she said. "I just don't have anything to give him. I don't want him to feel like I'm his responsibility. You don't know what it's like to see something you want more than your next breath and know you don't deserve to have it."

Her face told Job that Christy was speaking from her heart. Her visible emotions were very like Gabriel's. He hesitated and then pointed toward the river. "He'll be down there by the picnic grounds. I don't know what he'll say, but I think you should tell him how you feel. He thinks you've been blowing him off."

Gabe wished he had gone running instead of walking. He felt strangely energized in the midst of being horribly depressed. He wondered if the blood pressure medicine was responsible for the feeling that he had an unlimited reserve that morning. He tried to focus on the success of controlling his blood pressure, but his mind kept drifting back to Christy and what he had wanted more than anything else.

Walking alone seemed to amplify his loss of direction. It was too early for tourists to be in the park. He looped the path once and sat down on a bench to pray. He was very focused on his prayer but still came to his feet when he heard someone approaching. It was Christy. She smiled on seeing him.

"I missed you," she said. "Job thought you would be down here." She had wanted to say more, but Gabe's face gave her little encouragement.

"He knows me really well," Gabe said. "This is my running route." He glanced at his watch. "I guess we should head to the college."

"Do I look good enough to sit in on your class?" she asked. "I'm not scientifically gifted, but I'd like to hear you teach."

"You look fine," he said. He was trying not to make eye contact. Looking at her filled him with longing. "I have to go to Asheville this afternoon. It's a long drive. You might want to stay with Reba and Jonah. I could take you there after my classes."

"Could I go with you?" she begged. "I thought we could talk. What do you have to do there?"

"I have a meeting," he said. He thought he didn't want something he was battling to accept to be the topic of conversation. They had almost reached his truck when he decided that he had asked Christy to commit her life to him. He felt her answer had clearly been negative, but he thought telling her about his diagnosis would make it easier for both of them to walk away. He expected her response to be different.

"I'm going to the VA Hospital. I'm starting to develop diabetes. I found out on Monday, and I haven't really got my head straight about it yet. I thought I could avoid it, but you can't change your past indiscretions or your gene pool."

"It must be hard for you," she said. "You tried so hard to be healthy."

"I watched diabetes kill my mother. I've come to think she wanted it to take her life, but that's another long story." He unlocked the truck door and held it open for Christy. "It was a big shock, but I can handle it. I'm just on the learning curve right now. I'm going to Asheville to meet with the diabetes educator. I don't think you'd find that very interesting."

"If you still want me in your life, I should probably know about how to help you." Christy knew Gabe was still keeping distance between them because she had hurt him. She had stated her longing to be with him as plainly as she could, but she had to wait for his answer until he climbed into the truck beside her. He didn't answer the way she had hoped he would.

"We'll get some lunch before we leave. My class will finish at noon." There was no emotional response in his words.

It was a quiet ride. Gabe was feeling very unfocused and spent the drive going over his lecture in his mind. Christy spent the time feeling lost. She wondered if Job Killian had been right in thinking she should just leave. By the time they reached the college, she was near tears.

They arrived at the biology lab at nine o'clock. The room was already filled with students bearing numerous sample bottles. They were all near Christy's age, and she blushed when she saw several of them glance surreptitiously in her direction. She wondered if the attention would embarrass Gabe, but he showed no signs of noticing it. He moved to the front of the classroom and began giving his students instructions. He didn't make eye contact with Christy during the class. He didn't even look in her direction.

"If you guys followed directions as well as you usually do, you should have seven different water samples from the Deep Creek Campground. What you're going to do today is analyze them for bacterial counts, particularly coliforms, which you don't want to drink in large quantities for obvious reasons. Since David was also efficient, I have seven samples up here that I'm going to analyze and compare my results with your results. Don't throw out your samples when you finish because next Wednesday we'll be analyzing the mineral content and then screening it for heavy metal and hydrocarbon contaminants. Let's get started."

Christy sat at an empty desk and watched as Gabe showed them how to do bacterial counts. He did his at the microscope in front of the class in less than an hour and then circulated through the room checking results. She felt even more inadequate when she saw some of the girls looking up at him adoringly. They looked younger and prettier than she was. They weren't wearing baggy sweat clothes, and they looked as if their whole lives were still before them. Christy thought her life might really be over because she had hesitated to accept Gabriel Killian's offer.

When all the students had tabulated their results, Gabe displayed his own counts and discussed the reasons for their errors and why the counts were so important.

"I think you can all see why you need to boil ground water when you're out in the woods. Your essay question for next week's class is how did people survive drinking contaminated water for thousands of years, and how do they survive it now in third world countries? Be ready to discuss how the mineral content varies in water and why. You need to know the difference between hard and soft water. You might want to look at the materials on water sources in the western United States. There will be serious extra credit for anyone who finds out why some western water sources don't contain any visible life forms."

There were questions for several minutes. Christy had never really found science interesting until she had watched Gabe teach. He seemed to be gifted in so many ways that she felt even less adequate to be in his life. She knew he wouldn't suffer for company if she weren't around, but the thought of not being with him was unbearable. She spent the rest of the class agonizing about how she could remove the barriers she had created between them.

When the class had dispersed, Gabe checked to make sure all the equipment was cleaned and stored before putting his water samples in the refrigerator.

"That's it," he said. "Let's go." He couldn't keep the reluctance from his voice.

He put his computer bag over his shoulder and held the door for Christy. He didn't touch her even when she let her hand brush his invitingly. She knew she had driven him away by the time they reached his truck. She remembered Reba's warning and was certain she had done everything wrong in their relationship. She thought she should leave before she made his pain even greater because she didn't want the guilt of knowing she had destroyed his life. Her own life was over. It had been over for years.

When Gabe got into the truck she said, "Just leave me at the bus station. It will be better for us if I go." The words hit Gabe in the gut.

"Is that what you want?" he asked. It was a struggle to keep his emotions from coming out in those five words, but he was successful in convincing Christy that he didn't care. She burst into tears in response and got out of the truck.

"I can walk," she sobbed. "I don't want to put you to any more trouble. Thank you for everything."

Gabe crossed the seat immediately and exited Christy's door to pursue her. He caught her twenty yards from the truck and put his arms around her. She had intended to hold herself stiffly until he released her. She couldn't. Her face was wet when she pressed it against his jacket. His grasp told her what she couldn't see on his face. She clung to that feeling with desperation.

"I'm in love with you," she sobbed. "I love you, Gabriel. Please forgive me. I would do anything to make you feel like you did before all this happened I thought it would be better for you if I left, but I can't stand it. I feel like I'll die if I can't be with you."

He closed his eyes and held her even more tightly. He wanted to believe her, but he also felt like running away from the two days of mixed messages she had given him. He pushed all his reservations aside because he couldn't bear to lose even a chance to be with her. An inner strength that came as an answer to his prayer helped him push the past from his mind.

"I want to believe you, Christy. I need to believe this could happen in my life especially now, but I'm afraid of being wrong about our feelings. At first you made me feel like I've never felt before, but since Tuesday you've hit every vulnerable place in my heart. If we are meant to be together, you'll have to learn to deal with the scars of my past just like I'll have to deal with yours. Let's get away from here and talk."

She got into the truck, but she was still crying silently as they drove toward the interstate. His words had confirmed what she had sensed. She didn't really believe any words could take them past her mistakes. They were ten miles down the interstate before Gabe could think of what he needed to say.

"I believe everything you told me, and I know how it is to live in fear, Christy. I can't know how scared you are, but I know how it is to be helpless at someone else's mercy. I can't remember a day when I wasn't afraid until I was six. My stepfather was abusive, but it wasn't just verbal abuse. He beat me until he broke my bones. I wasn't even two years old when it started, but I can still remember every minute I spent at his mercy. No one came to my rescue until I hated everyone because no one cared how much I suffered. One night my mother was afraid he would kill me, and she shot him. She went to prison for saving my life. It wasn't right that it happened, but it happened. The one thing I took away from eleven years of counseling is that nobody can ever make it go away. You just have to go on. The worst part is having problems with feeling vulnerable. Because I feel that way, I've never let anyone get close to me outside of Jonah, Reba, Job, and a few guys I served with in the Navy.

"I think I fear getting close to people because I never could get close to my mother after she went to prison. We were very close before that, but she believed being in prison would dishonor me so she pushed me away. Even when she needed me to take care of her, she wouldn't let me do it. I think she thought she was doing me a favor, but she hurt me more than any beating ever did.

"I left home when I was seventeen and didn't come home for more than a visit until I was hurt. My mother had developed diabetes when she was twenty-eight, but I didn't know until I came home from the Navy. She was losing her vision by then. I had to take her to the doctor because she couldn't see well enough to drive. She was going blind from the diabetes, and they told us the only way to stop the eye disease was for her to keep her blood sugar around 100. Every time they checked her blood sugar it would be 300. Anything over 140 is abnormal. I came home and counted her medicine. It was obvious she wasn't taking it. I started giving her

pills and insulin to her and testing her sugars with the
machine she had but didn't use. I asked her to take care
of herself for my sake. I never saw any evidence that she
did. When I was controlling the medicine, she just ate
everything she wasn't supposed to have. I'd confront
her over eating candy, and she told me it was the only
thing that gave her any pleasure.

"Everything she did made me more frustrated until
I didn't want to see her at all. I've had to pray for forgiveness for how I felt because I shouldn't have let her
push me away. Even when she was dying, we couldn't
talk. She had a heart attack when I was at UNC doing
my graduate work. She died after I got to the hospital.
I sat with her and held her hand, but neither of us said
anything. She was looking at me when she died.

"Ever since then I've felt really guilty for not making her talk. When I was a kid, it was her fault. When
we were both adults, the blame has to go both ways.
If I had ever told her that I loved her and understood
why, I think we could have talked. But maybe even that
wouldn't have been enough. I'll never know now. The
Bible says love never fails, but it did. I know the Bible
isn't ever wrong, so I have to believe she and I caused it
to fail. I don't think I would have it in me to try to trust
and love another person if it weren't for Jonah, Reba,
Naomi, and Job.

"I don't like being alone, but I think I had subcon-
sciously chosen to be alone until I met you. From the
first time we went out, I felt like you understood me in
ways no one else ever has. I guess I need someone more
than I wanted to. I know that I love the person I believe
you are, but I couldn't handle being wrong about this,
Christy. I don't want you to go, but I can't live with feeling like you aren't sure. If you aren't completely sure
about being with me, please don't make me believe it's
possible again."

He could feel her eyes on him and glanced at her to try and read her thoughts. She spoke as he did.

"Until the night I ran away from the compound, the worst day of my life was when my grandmother was buried. I was standing next to her coffin when I just lost it. I couldn't stop crying so I went to stand behind a big potted plant. I heard my grandmother's best friends talking. They said I was the reason she died. They said it had been too much of a strain on her to take care of me. I knew they were right. I had been a terrible burden on her. My parents didn't leave enough money to take care of me. She had gone back to work to support me. For a long time I wished I had died with my parents. I don't ever want to be responsible for someone I love dying for me. I'm just not worth that risk."

All the negative feelings in Gabe's heart dissipated with her words. He knew she had only pushed him away to protect him.

"I think when two people love each other, they're in this world to stand behind each other. If that meant I died to protect you and our children, I'd see that as a good reason to give my life."

"I want to live for you," she whispered. "I want you to live for me. Do you still want to marry me?"

"I really do," he said. "I think you need to realize that I might be a burden on you at some point. Diabetes can be a terrible disease. I can promise that I'll try not to let it make me sick, but I can't promise it won't affect our life."

"I don't care," she said. "I want to take care of you. It's not because I want to repay you. I think you're supposed to take care of the people you love."

"It's ironic," he said. "We almost let bad communication keep us apart. I think one of my best memories is the night we laid in the back yard and looked at the stars. I'd like to feel that close to you for the rest of my life."

She unfastened her seat belt and slid into the middle seat. She took his hand and held it tightly. "I want to give you forever."

He put his arm around her shoulders and smiled. He let himself hope that he was reading her intentions right and released his reservations. "It's really hard to drive when all you want to do is let your feelings go." He felt like holding his breath when he asked the question and knew she would know what he meant if they were meant to be together. "Did you bring your driver's license?"

"Yes," she said. "Let's get married. I want to belong to you." Gabe answered by pulling his truck off the road and pulling her into his arms.

CHAPTER 12

Everything seemed simple during the remainder of the two-hour drive. They stopped at a fast food restaurant and bought grilled chicken sandwiches before getting back on the interstate to drive to Asheville. Gabe went to a hotel first and reserved a room. He asked the concierge for the address of the nearest wedding chapel and called to make a reservation for a six o'clock ceremony. They hurried to city hall and bought a license. It was a rushed transaction so they could make Gabriel's appointment with Mr. Bodine. They both forgot that Christy's identity would be in a public document. The document also connected Christy's name with Gabe's address. The license was being registered into the state's data bank as they left the building. In Tennessee a computer program picked up Christy's name and social security number and began alarming.

The educator met them in the waiting room. It was the first time Gabe had really looked at the fellow diabetic. Bodine was slightly overweight and carried the excess around his middle, but he didn't look as unhealthy as many of the non diabetics Gabe knew.

"I was afraid you might not show," Bodine said. "They blew you away on Monday, didn't they? I remember how I felt when they told me. It's like being a deer in the headlights."

"I assumed I could keep from getting it," Gabe said. "I hadn't ever thought about what I would do if I had it. I've started feeling better about living with it today." He was startled to realize that was the truth. He pulled Christy forward. "This is my fiancée, Christy. I wanted her to come."

"It's good to meet you, Christy." Mr. Bodine led them to a classroom and closed the door. When they were seated, he pulled out a big chart and taught them about insulin and how it was made by beta islet cells in the pancreas. The chart told them insulin was supposed to control how the body burns its main fuel, glucose. Insulin's other function was controlling growth factors that were designed to repair injuries to all parts of the body.

"You inherit resistance to the glucose effects only. When you make more insulin to keep your blood sugar down, you also get too much of the growth factor effects. For that reason, you really need to keep your body from needing insulin to control your blood sugar. You shouldn't eat if you aren't hungry."

"I've been doing that since I left the Navy," Gabe said. "It's too easy for me to gain weight otherwise."

"Go light on breakfast or don't eat breakfast at all," Mr. Bodine advised. "Your body is very resistant to the glucose effects of insulin in the morning, and your body makes sugar all night when you're asleep. If you eat in the morning, it's like topping off a full gas tank. It's almost impossible for your body to control your blood sugar after breakfast."

"I don't usually eat breakfast," Gabe said. "I drink tea, but I use artificial sweetener."

"That's good," Mr. Bodine said. He displayed a chart of foods. These are carbohydrates. He indicated fruit, table sugar, rice, pasta, bread, root vegetables like potatoes and tomato sauce and paste.

"Why are tomatoes a carbohydrate?" Christy asked.

"They're a fruit. When you cook them down into sauce or paste, you make tomato jam." Mr. Bodine passed her a cookbook. "This has tips on how to modify your recipes. Mr. Killian shouldn't eat these foods unless he's going to be very active. They are fast body fuels. The only other danger foods are saturated fats. Those are mainly animal fats. They make a normal person resistant to insulin for four hours after they are eaten. The worse possible combination you can eat is fat and carbohydrates."

"That's fast food," said Christy. "What should he eat? I want to help him stay healthy."

Gabe had still feared Christy might be frightened away by the prospects of life with diabetes. As she leaned over the food chart, he knew she didn't fear diabetes and was ready to fight it with him. It was a reassurance.

"He needs to eat fruits and vegetables with as much fiber as possible so you want them steamed or blanched," Bodine continued. "The more fiber you leave, the fewer calories he'll absorb. He can have lean cuts of meat in small quantities and low fat dairy products. The amount of calories he needs will vary with how active he is. The total amount of carbohydrates is actually more important to your blood sugar and weight than the kind of carbo-hydrate. If he runs an hour every night, he'll burn about two hundred calories, which is the equivalent of three slices of bread. He's close to ideal body weight now. We want him to achieve and maintain ideal body weight with the same or more muscle mass."

"I eat twice as much as he does," Christy said.

"You're lucky," Mr. Bodine said. "You can enjoy your food without guilt for now. A hundred years ago, you might have starved to death in times of famine. The ability to hold weight while being starved probably kept Native American people alive during drastic changes in climate. Nature selected a gene pool of slow metabolizers." He looked at Gabe. "Your body doesn't make insulin normally for the first thirty minutes after you eat. You need to get up and exercise the second you finish eating. That lets your muscles use the sugar you've eaten without needing insulin. Then you test your sugar one hour after you eat. If you have the right combination of food and exercise, you can keep your sugar under 140. If you keep your sugar down, you won't get eye or kidney disease. The medications you're taking are protecting you from heart disease."

"Is diabetes in your family?" Gabe asked.

"My father died from it," said the educator. "He had the 'eat, drink and be merry for tomorrow you will die anyway' philosophy. Often people get that form of cynicism when they've watched people they love die from diabetes. Don't go there. Diabetes doesn't have to be a disease. It isn't for me. I can't promise you eternal health, but I haven't developed any signs of damage, and I've had it almost nine years." He took out his meter and did a blood sugar at the same time as Gabe. Gabe's reading was 157 to Bodine's 112.

"Fast food did that," said Christy. "We can't eat that anymore. We'll just bring food with us."

"How can I keep my islet cells from failing?" Gabe asked. "I thought I could avoid this with diet and exercise, but it was obviously too little too late. I guess I have what they call borderline diabetes, and I don't want it to get worse."

"You have type 2 diabetes, Mr. Killian. There is no borderline. In my opinion, we ought to lower the sugar level where we diagnose diabetes. You failed your glucose tolerance test so you don't have the denial option of impaired glucose tolerance. Your fasting sugar was only 124, but the one and two hour sugars after you drank glucose solution were over 200. We see that frequently in ethnic populations like Native Americans. As for your lifestyle modification, you did avoid diabetes for a long time. Most of your generation is developing diabetes ten years earlier than their parents did. You didn't know about the risk early enough to avoid sugar and fat in your childhood and twenties, but your lifestyle kept you from developing it in your twenties. We try to target high risk children now. When you have kids, they need to follow this same diet. The epidemic of diabetes in America came when we started eating sugar and fat without exercising. There are children with type 2 diabetes now. That's the trend we must stop.

"To answer your question, the drugs in the thia-zoli-dinedione class seem to protect your islet cells and your ability to make insulin. I'm on one of them. It's called Avandia. I've been on it for the last two years. Before Avandia, I was on the maximal dose of two other pills with insulin at night. Now I take Avandia and metfor-min. Metformin is another insulin sensitizing drug. It keeps your liver from making sugar when you've eaten. It works really well in overweight people like me. I only need insulin when I'm ill or really cheating on my diet. When you come back for your next clinic visit, talk to your doctor about insulin sensitizing drugs. No other medicines prevent islet cell failure. That's why most non insulin dependent diabetics end up taking insulin."

They talked about having yearly eye checks to look for cataracts and blood vessel damage, and they talked about checking the amount of microscopic albumen in Gabe's urine every year to check for kidney disease. "That was done on Monday," Mr. Bodine said. "You don't have any sign of kidney disease. You are at more risk since your mother had kidney disease, and being on the ACE inhibiting blood pressure medicine protects your kidneys. You need to keep your pressure under 130/80 all the time."

"I've been checking," Gabe said. "Can my blood pressure go too low?"

"ACE inhibiting drugs and ARB drugs don't keep your body from reacting to a low blood pressure like some of the older blood pressure medicines. If your blood pressure does drop, you'll feel dizzy or light headed, and your pulse will speed up. If you don't feel any symptoms, your pressure isn't too low no matter what it reads. The same goes for your blood sugar.

"The ACE drugs have two major side effects. One is a dry cough. If you have spells of coughing when you aren't sick with a cold or allergies, let us know. The other complication is called angioneurotic edema. You get an area of swelling as if you had been stung by a bee or wasp. If you develop that, it's an emergency. You need to get to a hospital immediately."

"No other side effects?" Gabe asked hesitantly. "I've heard stories about other problems."

"Not with these drugs," Bodine said. "That's one reason why we use them. Other types of blood pressure medications can have sexual side effects, but these drugs don't usually cause a problem. I take one, and I'd definitely be complaining if they did. What most men don't realize is that sick blood vessels cause sexual problems. If you keep all your risk factors for heart disease in line, you shouldn't ever have sexual problems either."

The session ended at five o'clock. As they were leaving, Gabe remembered to ask for enough samples of the two pills to hold him until they returned to Cherokee. Christy went to the bathroom, giving Gabe the chance to ask Bodine the question he needed answered.

"I want to marry Christy and have a family. I keep thinking it isn't fair to put this on her and our children."

"Then don't let it hurt you," Bodine said. "You're lucky. You have time to fight back. If you need moral support, give me a call." He put his card into Gabe's hand and left him. Gabe felt calm for the first time since he had heard the diagnosis. In the truck, he put his hands on Christy's face and looked into her eyes.

"Are you sure about getting married? This is your last chance to back out, and I'd understand if you wanted to."

"You'll have to come up with a lot better reason than diabetes," she said. "It doesn't scare me."

He looked into her eyes and thought of the differences in their backgrounds. "One last question. Being a Native American isn't something I am. It's who I am and the way I live. I couldn't ever leave that way of life, and I want my children to be Cherokee even if they're only half Cherokee by blood. Will you be okay with that?"

"I love you," she said. "I love everything you are. I wouldn't want you to be any different. I want our children to be just like you." She put her arms around him and kissed him without holding back any of her feelings. Within minutes, both of them were lost in the need to make love. Gabe broke away and put his key in the ignition.

"Marriage first. Keep saying that while I drive."

They had time to stop at a mall and buy Christy two dresses, a pant suit, and a pair of sandals. Gabe also bought her a shawl although Christy didn't understand why until later. He bought two changes of clothes for himself while she used her sixty four dollars to buy Gabe a narrow gold wedding band. He spent considerably more on her wedding band and hid it from her as they left the store.

The preacher's wife was a diminutive gray-haired lady who doubled as the musician. She was beaming when she met them in the foyer and took Christy to change. Gabe paid for the service and then waited for his bride with sudden anxiety. He found himself fearing she might change her mind at the last minute and prayed he was wrong.

"Don't fret," the elderly preacher reassured him. "When they sign the license, they always show up for the ceremony. This must be your first marriage."

"And last," Gabe asserted. "For both of us."

"Now I won't be anxious for you," the preacher said.

Gabe reached for the preacher's Bible and flipped the pages rapidly to I Corinthians. He pointed to the thirteenth chapter and asked, "Could you read this in the ceremony?"

"I would be happy to read it," the preacher replied.

Gabe extended the white shawl to the preacher. "If you could use this at the end, it would make the ceremony mean even more to us. I'm Cherokee. This part of the old ways is important to me."

"I've seen more than a few ceremonies with the shawl," the preacher said. "I'll see that you get properly hitched before you leave here." They both turned as the musician cleared her throat and then took her seat at the organ. When she began playing, Christy walked down the aisle slowly to strains of the wedding march. She kept her eyes on the floor until she reached Gabriel's side and felt him take both her hands. When she looked up at him with love on her face, he knew his fears were groundless. He held her hands tightly as the minister read the words in I Corinthians 13.

"Love suffereth long and is kind. Love envieth not. Love vaunteth not itself and is not puffed up. Doth not behave itself unseemly. Seeketh not her own. Is not easily provoked. Thinketh no evil. Rejoiceth not in iniquity, but rejoiceth in the truth. Beareth all things, believeth all things, hopeth all things, endureth all things. Love never faileth."

The passage was Christy's favorite. She knew without asking that Gabe had chosen it. In having the preacher say those words, he was putting the past behind him. It sealed the feeling that they had been brought together by God. Christy was smiling through her tears when they took the vows. It moved her to feel Gabe's unsteady hands slip a beautiful gold ring on her hand. It was carved in the shape of gold leaves woven in a circle. She had never seen another wedding band like it. She thought it was perfect.

She was looking into Gabriel's dark eyes and feeling as if they were alone on earth when the minister said, "I now pronounce you man and wife." He put the shawl around both of them and tied the ends together loosely. Gabe pulled Christy even closer.

"You're my wife in every way now." When Gabe kissed her, Christy wrapped her arms around him tightly and didn't want to let him go.

The musician witnessed their license and took a series of pictures before they took their leave. Gabe wrapped the white, silk shawl around his bride as they left the chapel. In the truck, Christy slid across the seat so she could put her arms around Gabe.

"Tell me about the shawl."

"In traditional Cherokee weddings, a blanket or shawl is tied around the bride and groom. It signifies how your lives are tied together by being married."

"They couldn't tie me close enough," Christy said. When Gabe kissed her, she allowed herself to touch him without the boundaries they had set before their wedding. She could feel how much he wanted her in his response.

"We need to go to the hotel before we get arrested for making love in the parking lot," he said. "Do you want to get something to eat first?"

"I was thinking about room service later tonight," Christy said. "I was thinking about being with you now."

She kissed him again and let her hand run over his chest. The touch persuaded her husband to go to the hotel.

In the elevator, Gabe had a renewed anxiety attack about diabetes and blood pressure medicine and what might happen when they made love. When they were alone between the fifth and tenth floors, Christy put her arms around him and began caressing his body. Her mouth brushed his cheek and followed her fingers to his mouth. They missed their floor once and barely managed to catch the door a second time. Christy pulled her husband to their room door and clung to him as he fumbled with the key. They fell in the door onto the soft carpet. Christy was laughing as she kicked the door shut.

"That wasn't graceful, but I couldn't wait any longer to be close to you." She leaned over Gabe's body to look into his eyes. He could feel the caress of her breath on his face when she whispered, "I love you, Gabriel. I will always love you."

The words made him want her more. He caught her hair in his hand and pushed her back on the carpet. He knew she hadn't ever been with a man, but Christy seemed as eager to make love as he was. She removed his jacket and then hesitated as her hands found the holster. He released her long enough to remove it and then realized the one thing they had overlooked.

"We forgot about birth control, Christy."

"I don't care unless you do," she said fervently. "I wouldn't care if I knew we were making a baby tonight. I love you, and I don't want anything coming between us."

He felt her lips against his neck and her hands on his chest as if those sensations could suppress every other sensation in his body. Christy could feel his breath quicken and unbuttoned his shirt rapidly. She kissed the bare skin of his chest as she pulled his tie free.

"I want to be joined with you, Gabe." He pulled her tightly into his arms and kissed her as she trembled.

"I hope we are making a baby, Christy," he whispered. He left only her silk slip between them until even that filmy fabric seemed too intrusive. Inexperience was never a barrier. They were both so caught up in passion that every touch and move seemed perfect.

Gabe did make a tremendous effort to move slowly and gently because he wanted her to know the act was for both of them. He hadn't expected to feel like he was making love for the first time. The almost buried memory of peer pressure sex wasn't anything like making love with his wife. Her inexperienced hands made him feel more desire than he had believed possible. The waiting to make her pleasure greater was almost torture and yet he didn't want it to end. There was a moment when he felt as if their souls were as entwined as their bodies. Then he felt an emotional rush that had never been and could not ever be equaled. He had never felt so completely joined to another person. He thought he could have held her in his arms forever.

Gabe rolled onto his back and pulled Christy to lie on top of his body. She rested her chin on her folded hands and looked down into his eyes. Her face was soft, and even her eyes were smiling.

"I love you, Christy," he said. "I don't have the words to tell you how you make me feel."

"You made everything perfect," she whispered. "You make me so happy."

"You make me feel like I've found the missing half of life." He kissed her hair and held her so close that they could feel each other breathing. For the first time in his life, he felt as if he had found the whole scope of his destiny.

Gabriel carried Christy to the bed. They kept touching each other until heated desire was between them again. They made love even more slowly before sleeping in each other's arms. Neither of them ever remembered to call room service.

CHAPTER 13

Morning came and hours passed before Gabe awakened. Joy and relief had allowed him to relax for the first time in days, and he slept deeply until a distant sound startled him. He had a moment of panic when he heard the room door close. His fear intensified when he sat up and looked for Christy but didn't see her.

"Christy?"

"I'll be right there." She appeared wearing his shirt, which hung to her thighs. She was wheeling a room service cart.

"You've got to be hungry now, Gabriel. We both burned some serious calories." He laughed with relief and lay back as she sat down on the bed beside him. It intensified the feeling that she was a part of him to see her wearing his clothes.

"What time is it anyway?"

"Ten o'clock." She turned on the bedside lamp and offered him a strawberry from the cart. When he took it, she caressed his shoulders and chest marveling at how white her skin looked against his.

"How much Cherokee are you?"

"One hundred percent as far as I know. It's a big deal to know your quantum of blood when you live on the reservation."

"I want to know more about your life," she said. "I knew your heritage was important to you even before you told me yesterday."

"And how do you know that?" he asked.

"The eagle feather." She smiled at his expression. "I know you. Someday that won't surprise you." Her fingers stopped at the broad scar just under his left collarbone. "Is this where you were shot?"

"A little lower and I wouldn't be here." He pulled her close to kiss her lovingly. "I never thought it could have been a stroke of luck. If it hadn't happened, I'd still be in the Navy and I wouldn't have met you."

"Last night I kept thinking the same thing. If I hadn't been kidnapped, I wouldn't have come to Bryson City. It was worth everything to have met you."

In the afternoon, while Christy was sleeping close beside him, Gabe remembered his family. He had absolutely no regrets about marrying Christy, but he decided to give his family advance warning so only he would hear their reservations. He dressed and took his medication. Then he went to the living room to call Jonah and Reba. He reached his aunt, and she responded.

"Job told me you didn't come home last night. I guess congratulations are in order."

"I'm sure it was the right thing to do," Gabe said. "I know it was sudden, and I know we haven't known each other long, but Reba, I'm sure she's the one. Tell Jonah we talked about everything present, past, and future. We'll be home tomorrow night. Will you tell Job and explain to Jonah for me?"

"Jonah wants you to be happy, Gabe," Reba said gently. "If you're happy with this, we'll be happy for you. I'll tell Job. Tell Christy we're glad to have her in the family."

Gabe heaved a sigh of relief when he hung up the phone, and then he flipped through the local attraction magazine provided by the hotel looking for some place special to take his bride.

He awakened his Christy by kissing her ear. "Time for supper, Mrs. Killian." Christy rolled over slowly and put her arms around him. She felt rested and ready to face the world for the first time in almost two years.

"You're dressed," she observed. "I'm disappointed."

"I want to take you out tonight," Gabe said. "I've found something in town that I think you'll really like. This will also give you something you can tell people we did on our honeymoon." He showed her his watch. "You've got twenty minutes until our reservation for supper. The show we're going to starts at seven."

Christy was having a good time, and it was an alien, wondrous feeling. She dressed in her sun dress and left her hair loose on her shoulders because she knew her husband liked it that way. They took the stairs to the lobby level and walked to a nearby restaurant without Gabe suggesting it. During the walk, Christy said, "We should walk everywhere. Cars are part of the problem."

"I think no activity is some of it," Gabe said. "I think being human garbage disposals is the rest of it. You don't have to give up the things you like because of me. I have reasonable self control."

"I want to eat the right way," she said. "When we have kids, they will need to stay away from sugar and junk food. It will be better for all of us if it isn't in the house. The only thing I'll miss is chocolate, but I can live without it."

"I don't like chocolate," Gabe said. "Maybe I'll buy you some as a reward for being the perfect wife."

They had supper while Christy tried to get Gabe to tell her where they were going and left to walk around the city to burn off the meal. Despite Christy's constant

attempt to learn their destination, Gabe didn't waiver
in his effort to surprise her. He kept diverting her with
conversation until they were walking into the civic center.
Their tickets told her they would be seeing a Cherokee
dance troupe.

Christy was awe inspired by the art form she had
never seen. Gabe whispered to her about the various
dances as they watched dancers as young as five per-
form the grass dance. Each age group seemed to have
a deeper knowledge of the steps and the emotions they
were meant to portray. She could scarcely contain her
questions until they were outside again.

"Do you know how to do those dances, Gabriel?"

"Not very well. I have a friend in Cherokee who
dances in shows and competitions all over the southeast,
but it's something you really have to work at. Zack has
been doing it all his life. It's sort of a tradition in his family. The people who really do it right start teaching the
children when they're four or five. They learn the grass
dance because that was the dance that flattened the grass
in a new campsite before the other dancers performed.
They always make a circle.

"I didn't come back to North Carolina until I was
almost seven, and then it was a long time before I felt
like I belonged enough to get involved with the tribe. A
boy has his parents' identity until he's a man, and my
father was dead. My mother wasn't with me. In all the
ways that matter, Jonah and Reba are my parents. They
had other things that they considered more important
than dancing."

"Why weren't there any women dancing?" she
asked.

"The dances can have men or women, which is
something distinctive about the Cherokee. When women
dance with the men, they follow the lead dancer. Don't
think women aren't important in Cherokee society. They
have their own dances that don't include any men. The

original seven Cherokee clans were passed along the maternal line. If I had married two hundred years ago, I would have left my clan and family and gone to live with my wife's family. It was the law that you had to marry out of your clan. I think I've definitely done that."

"What were the dances done for?"

"They were worship," Gabe said. "They were done to ask the supreme being for a good hunt or to give thanks for a good harvest. We were always a monotheistic people so we were easily converted to Christianity. The most technical dance is the Eagle Dance. That's the only time the Cherokee used feathers except in the capes the chiefs wore and the two feathers in our hair."

"I want to paint what it would have looked like then," she said wistfully. She turned around and walked backwards looking at him. "Gabriel, you can be my model."

"Hey, I've heard about artists' models," he said. "My position on that is I get full right of approval on how undressed you make me. I've got to be able to teach without having everybody in the room giggling."

"How do you know they would giggle? I didn't giggle." She stopped him from walking and stood on her tiptoes to kiss him. "I want your approval, and I'm too jealous to let anybody else see how good you really look."

His eyes told her that she was saying the right words. She took his hand and made him hurry up the hill to their hotel. That night she felt as if she couldn't get him close enough.

"The hard part about this will be leaving tomorrow," Christy whispered. "I like having you all to myself." She shivered as Gabe ran his hands over her bare shoulders and back.

"You're my priority," he told her. "All my time doing other things will be to make our life better. I feel like I could do absolutely anything today. It's a major rush compared to the last week."

"That was my fault," Christy said soberly. "I'm just glad you could forgive me." She sighed and rested her head on his shoulder. "Mr. Bodine made you feel better, didn't he?"

"Better than the books. Everything I read overwhelmed me. They don't put those books together really well. They put everything that scares you in the first chapter. They give it to you when you don't feel ready to try and control diabetes. Then they tell you controlling it is your only hope. Last Monday I had the feeling they thought I would already know what I needed to do because my mother had it or because I'm a biologist. I'm a marine biologist. If fish had it, I'd know about it. Actually catfish might. They eat garbage, too.

"I found out that I was ready to *prevent* it and not to *have* it. I didn't read anything about it when my mother was sick. I learned what medicine to give her and how to give insulin shots. I learned how to test her blood sugar. I didn't want to know more because it scared me."

"Are you scared now?" she asked.

"Yes, but I have an objective. I want to live with you for the next fifty or sixty years and prove to everyone in Cherokee that this isn't a death sentence. I believe I can do it because I have you. My grandfather always said every man has things he fears. All you can do is pray for God to give you a strong heart so you can defeat them. I think God gave you to me so I could have a strong heart."

"I think you had it all along," she said seriously. "I could feel that spirit in you. It makes me feel like we can do anything." She smiled suddenly. "That would have been your name, Gabriel. Like you said before about Native Americans taking a name that described something about them. Your name would have been 'Strong Heart.'"

The words were a confirmation that she understood his life and the way he wanted to live. "I think our family name would have been Strongheart. I never felt as strong in spirit as I feel now." He pressed his right hand against her left hand, viewing the wedding ring with pleasure. She slid her fingers over his hand and up his arm feeling the bruise over his vein with surprise.

"What happened to your arm, Gabriel? Is this where they drew your blood at the VA?"

"That's on the other arm. This is the souvenir from when I donated blood for you. I have AB- blood, too. We can tell people we're blood siblings now. If you start getting really dark tans, you'll know why. You might only need sunscreen on the back of your neck."

"I have a confession to make," she said. "You never had any sunburn on your neck. I just wanted to talk to you, and I couldn't think of anything else to say."

"It was the best lie anyone ever told me." He pulled her head down and stroked her hair. "This is the first time since I left the Navy that I've felt like I was really going home."

CHAPTER 14

They left early enough Sunday to go to church service and then to the outlet mall. Gabe took great pleasure in buying Christy more clothes, though she protested about spending the money. As they drove slowly through the mountains, they stopped at a lookout and stood in the ever present wind. When Gabriel kissed Christy, it stirred her emotions like the wind stirred her hair. She shuddered as she embraced him.

"I'm scared, Gabriel. I've been hiding for such a long time. Do you think they'll find me?" The intensity of her fear should have warned him, but Gabe was feeling too euphoric to be concerned about anything.

"Don't worry about things that haven't happened, Christy. When I was stressing over the diabetes, Jonah told me only my fear could kill me. That's how you need to look at this. My friend in the sheriff's office has already talked to the FBI. They're ready to talk to you whenever you're ready. Until then, no one knows your real name except me and my family." She relaxed against him and closed her eyes.

"I know you're right. It's just been a nightmare. I didn't think God was hearing my prayers because I couldn't wake up."

"God always has a reason," he said. "I've battled those same thoughts, but I'm glad He made you wait so I could be a part of your answer."

"Will your family be okay about us being married?"

"I already called them," Gabe said. "They're happy about it. They love me. They'll love you. Be happy or I'll feel like I'm not doing my part in this marriage." He kissed her and led her to the truck.

"You worry too much," he suggested. "When we get home, I'm going to read Judges to you about the prophet Deborah. When the men were afraid to go to war, she led them. You, too, can be Deborah, Mrs. Killian. Just in surviving all alone I think you've earned the right to be called a warrior."

She believed him and wasn't afraid for the remainder of their journey home. They stopped at a restaurant in Maggie Valley and had lunch. Gabe had a salad with low fat dressing and avoided the bread. He checked his blood sugar two hours later and found it was 103.

"Maybe I'm getting the hang of this," he said.

They were both feeling good about all aspects of their lives until they drove into Gabe's driveway and saw the three police cars parked in the yard. Their flashing lights were like a strobe penetrating Christy's soul. Gabe was out of the truck running to the men before Christy could gather her wits.

When she could get on her feet, she stumbled to the porch before Gabe saw her. Lying on the living room floor was Job's girlfriend, Darla. There was a bullet hole in her temple. Job was on a stretcher being attended by two paramedics. Blood was everywhere. Christy felt as if she couldn't breathe and then couldn't draw enough air into her lungs. The world spun around her and she fainted.

She was in a place she could not recognize even when her vision cleared. "Gabriel," she said in terror. Hands held her on a hard surface and for a terrible moment she thought she was at the compound again.

"No!" she screamed. "Let go of me. Let me go!" Gabriel was beside her instantly and gathered her into his arms.

"I'm here, Christy. It's okay. You're okay." She clung to him and sobbed as the vision of Darla flashed across her mind.

"They found me, Gabriel. They thought she was me."

"We can't be sure," Gabe said. "If Job lives…" His voice broke, and she realized he was crying. Her protective, mothering instincts pushed her own fears aside as she held her husband.

"It isn't your fault. You couldn't know."

"I should have known," Gabe agonized. "I know a lot more about the evil in this world than you do. Christy, you've got to talk to the federal people."

"I can do it," she said to Gabe and the policewoman beside her. "I want to do it."

She was in the back of a police van. The local officers transported Gabe and Christy to their headquarters. The drive gave them ten minutes to gather their shattered emotions. They were escorted to a windowless central room at the jail to meet with the FBI agents Buddy had summoned. The encounter was tape recorded, and Christy was asked to take an oath to tell the truth as if she were in court.

"Mrs. Killian, we need as much detail as possible about your alleged abduction and captivity."

Under the table, Gabe squeezed her hand urging her to ignore the word alleged. Her voice was tremulous, but she told a very coherent story.

"I started at Tucker College in the fall of 1996. I was an art student, and I had a scholarship. The town is called Tucker, too, and beginning in the fall of 1996 they held a blood drive for a little girl named Sheila Marsdon. They said she had leukemia and a rare blood type, AB-. They blood tested everyone at the school and asked those of us who had the type if we would give blood. We all donated, and that was it until the spring when they did it again. It happened again in the fall of 1997, and I didn't want to give again because it hurt so much. I hate needles.

They brought this nurse that time. His name was Chuck Portman, and he brought that gas the dentists use so the needles wouldn't freak us out. I didn't mind it so much that time, and I volunteered again in the spring of 1998. That time when I woke up I wasn't at Tucker anymore. I was in a compound, and it was surrounded by twelve-foot chain-link fence with barbed wire on top like prison. There were nineteen other people, all from Tucker, but some of them had been there for a year. They kept us there to donate blood. They gave us shots to make us make more blood, and then they took plasma every week and blood every two weeks. We were never told why, but Chuck told me the night he helped me get away. At first we were drugged to keep us from running away, but after a while we were too weak to try.

"People disappeared every few months, and there were new people when the old ones were gone. Finally I had been there the longest, and I thought that meant they would let me go soon. They took me to give blood one afternoon, but when I woke up, Chuck told me I had to do everything he said or we would both die. There was a body in the bed beside me. It was a girl I had known, and she was dead. Before I could think of what was happening, Chuck was carrying me out of the building over his shoulder. He told me they had ordered him to take all of my blood until I was dead, and he said that was what had happened to the others. I was so scared that I started waking up, and he put me down to let me run with him. Someone must have seen us because they shot at us, and they hit Chuck in the back. I didn't know it was so bad until later." She swallowed hard and looked at Gabe with remembered panic.

"Go on," he urged her.

"He gave me his car keys and told me where to drive. I never really knew where we were, but he knew back roads and finally we made it to the interstate. We tried to stop at his house so we could call for help, but there were cars in his driveway. He gave me my ID and some money. He told me that I needed to run and keep running. I had to make sure my name and social security number wasn't ever entered into any computers. I didn't know he was dying. I just kept driving down I-40 East."

"Chuck said the compound was owned by a rich family named Divilbiss. They all had some sort of clotting problem so they needed blood and clotting factors from plasma. They were AB-. Chuck said they were afraid of getting AIDS and hepatitis, so they had been bringing people to the compound for a long time. The blood drives were designed to test us for diseases, and if we didn't show any signs of disease for eighteen months, they took us. If you got anemic, they just took all your blood and buried your body." Her voice broke, and Gabe put his arm around her.

"Part of abducting us was taking all our ID. Chuck took mine back before he helped me escape. I didn't know he was hurt that bad until he was dead. I left the car at a rest station and hitched a ride with a trucker. The rest station was near Knoxville."

"Do you know what day you abandoned the car?" one of the agents asked.

"It was September 30, 1998. I know because of a newspaper in the trucker's rig. I've been hiding ever since then." The agents looked grim.

"It's obvious that they're still looking for you. Miss Ravenwood and Mr. Killian appear to have been shot with a high powered sniper rifle. It looks like the shooter was targeting the occupants of the house. I don't think they saw anyone or anything until it was over. There isn't much way to protect yourself against that kind of attack. It's the kind of killing we see with organized crime. Until this investigation is complete, you should probably be in protective custody."

Christy stared at the men not really understanding what they were telling her. She turned to Gabe for his decision. Her husband's face was unreadable as he looked at her.

"What do you want to do, Christy?"

"Tell me what to do," she said.

"We'd rather help you get them," Gabe said. His basic distrust of the system and its ability to rescue victims had reached a whole new level while listening to the federal agents. "If that isn't an option, then we'll pass on the protective custody. I can take care of Christy."

"I can't recommend that course of action," the agent objected. "If she's right about the name, there's a Divilbiss family in the Mafia. Before this is over you may end up in the federal witness protection program."

"If it comes to that, we'll deal with it," Gabe said. "Until then, I'd rather be a hunter than prey. I will want protection when I teach my classes. I just have one regular class this summer and some independent study courses."

"We'll know more in the next couple of days," the lead agent said. He dismissed his partners with his eyes. Two of the agents left them alone with Buddy and the lead agent. Buddy closed the door.

"Your friend here told me you'd be a hard sell, Mr. Killian. He tells me you were in the Navy for several years. He says you were a Seal."

"I was a Seal for seven years, and I don't wear the uniform but I still practice the craft." Gabe's voice was quietly confident. "I know how to hide in this kind of situation, and I can make sure Christy knows how. In the meantime, let's be frank. I work for the government, too. An investigation is bull for we'll put it on the list. It would seem to me since you know these people are willing to kill, you'd find this compound, raid it, and make sure there are too many witnesses to kill them all. All this investigation will do is give them time to move everything."

"It isn't that simple," the agent said. "Legally we can't raid private property without probable cause."

"One innocent girl with a bullet in her head and my cousin with a bullet in his neck looks like probable enough cause to me." Gabe stood, unable to conceal his anger past that point. "The government used to send me to do a lot more for less obvious reasons. We're going to head out into the park. I'll check in with Buddy every few days, but other than that only God is going to know where we'll be. I'll meet you in time for my class every Wednesday. If you get ready to give these people what they deserve, I'll be happy to go with you. If any of them come after me, I'll radio you and let you know where to find the bodies." The agent had been trained to follow rules, but he almost laughed at Gabe's flagrant defiance.

"Do you want some protection until you get your gear?"

"I'd appreciate it." Gabe took Christy's hand and led her out of the jail via a tunnel into the city administration building. The agent drove them to Gabe's home in a bullet proof car.

Christy was numb, and she watched Gabriel as if he were a stranger while he loaded two backpacks and two bedrolls in the dark living room. He changed clothes in the bathroom and returned in camouflage. "I left you

another set of fatigues in the bathroom," he told his wife.
"Change into them and put your hair up under the hat.
There's some makeup on the sink. Use it to cover your
face, neck, and hands. Stay away from the window."

While she was in the bathroom, he took a smaller
bag of gear and tied it to his backpack.

"Is that what I think it is?" the agent asked.

"I think I'll take the fifth amendment on that one."
Gabe tossed him a radio. "The frequency is on the
back."

The agent jotted down the frequency and returned
the radio. "I'll set mine on the same band. My name is
Parker. I prefer Hawkeye."

"Windrunner," Gabe said shortly. "Can I trust you
or are you going to launch into that ninety-day wonder
for the good of the corps garbage?"

"You can trust me," Hawkeye said sharply. "If it
were my choice, we'd be on our way to that compound
tonight. If your wife can think of anything else to help
us pinpoint it..."

"We'll be working on it." Gabe extended his hand
to the man. When they shook hands, the agent's dry
palm and firm grip made Gabe believe he wouldn't be
betrayed. He went into the bathroom and found Christy
staring at the camouflage makeup. She was obviously
bewildered and would have been an easy target from
the window. He pulled her into the bedroom and made
her sit on the floor below the windows. He sat in front
of her and gently applied the camouflage to her face and
then her neck and hands.

"Hey, this is just war paint," he said reassuringly.
"You're a Cherokee wife now, and you've got to learn
about doing battle. Normally we're a peaceful tribe, but
even the Bible says there's a time to fight. It's time to
fight, Christy, and I'll teach you how." Her hands were
shaking, and when Gabe had finished covering them,
he pulled her into his arms.

"I'm going to take care of you, Christy. Do you believe me?"

"I do believe you." She bit her lip and closed her eyes for a moment. "You may have to tell me what to do until I can breathe again."

"I'll tell you everything you need to know until you know you can trust me."

"I trust you now," she whispered. "And I would die for you, Gabe. Please don't let them hurt you. I couldn't stand it if you were hurt because of me." He pressed his fingertips to her lips.

"We're in this together. We'll take care of each other. When we pray, God will do the rest." He kissed her and communicated all the reassurances she needed to hear in that gesture. When he released her, he put the camouflage makeup in her backpack. They left the house for Hawkeye's bulletproof car.

They were driven to Bryson City and released on the road to Deep Creek. Christy could barely see in the cloudy darkness, but Gabe moved quickly into the trees paralleling the road until they reached the river. When they reached her former home, she was shocked because the route had been so circuitous. Gabe entered first and made certain the emergency exit door would allow them an escape route, and then they made their bed in the back of the bus. Christy lay down as if she could stop her terrified racing thoughts and sleep. She was startled when she felt Gabe's arms pull her back against him.

"We took a vow, Christy, and part of it was for better or for worse. Maybe if we get the worse part done now, we won't have to do it anymore."

"Did you see your uncle?" she whispered. "Did they blame me?"

"I couldn't reach them," he said. He couldn't keep the emotion from his voice because he blamed himself. "They're in Knoxville at the regional trauma center. I know they don't blame us. You're a victim, too. Let's pray and then try to get some sleep. We need to get higher into the mountains before the sun gets up." He oth of them, and the words let the tension in her chest ease until she could sleep. Every time she awakened, she moved closer to Gabe and prayed he would be kept safe.

Gabe lay awake praying silently for Job, the rest of his family, and his wife's safety. While he prayed, the rest of his mind was focused on standing guard.

CHAPTER 15

Christy awakened abruptly when she realized Gabe was no longer behind her. When she started to speak, he was immediately beside her with his hand on her lips. He shook his head and indicated the exit with his eyes.

Christy looked at her sleeping bag, and he nodded toward it and her backpack. When she saw he was holding his gun, she knew they were in eminent danger, and she rolled the sleeping bag hurriedly. He went out the emergency exit silently in the half light. His hand summoned her to follow. They were deep into the kudzu-covered forest before he would even chance whispering to her.

"When the forest gets quiet, the two-legged animals are around. We need to get into that outcropping of rocks and take cover where we have an advantage."

He obviously expected obedience and not a response. Christy followed him over the roughest trail she had ever negotiated. Actually, it wasn't a trail as much as a path used by forest animals. She was certain Gabe intended to leave it as if no one had walked through it. More than two hours passed before they reached the rocks, and by then she was starving and tired. Gabe propelled her into a shallow cave and put his backpack at her feet. She was relieved to see the packets of dried fruit and homemade granola and thankful to eat one. Gabe disappeared to do his own reconnaissance and returned to eat his breakfast.

"I think we lost them. Our edge will be the terrain. Most assassins aren't going to be survivalists." She wanted to protest that her own survival skills were limited, but she just forced a smile.

"I'm glad you are. I just worry about you being up here when you're diabetic."

"Don't," he said. "We're going to live the way my people lived before diabetes was killing us. We're going to eat everything but processed foods, drink water, and burn every calorie we eat. I think this is exactly what I need to feel like I'm in control of my life. I brought my pills, my glucose meter, and my favorite form of exercise with me."

Christy relaxed. Knowing he could calm her made Gabriel feel more in control.

"I get the feeling we might be following the cloud in the wilderness," she said.

"That's the idea," he said. "We'll also be doing my job. Remember I told you that I also work for the National Park Service. We're going to be surveying. That's what I would have been doing every day except class days anyway. Hey, look at it this way. There are rich people who pay for this kind of adventure. You're about to have a seriously memorable honeymoon." She did smile then and moved closer to kiss him. It felt safe to make love with him, and she wanted to feel safe. Gabe responded to her touch eagerly for several moments and then held her.

"Hold that thought until tonight. We can't risk letting our guard down right now."

They stayed in the cave until ten o'clock and saw no signs they were being followed. When they left, they hiked upward staying on the rockiest ground and moving through dense underbrush. Christy came to appreciate the camouflage fatigues even though they were several sizes too large. The heavy material protected her legs and arms. She wondered why Gabe had clothes that were obviously too small for him and finally asked.

"Whose fatigues were these, Gabriel?"

"They were mine after Seal training," he laughed. "I weigh about 185 pounds now. When I finished the Seal training, I weighed 148. I looked like a toothpick. When I came home on leave, Reba insisted on feeding me because she thought they were killing me." He slowed his pace and took her hand. "When we get some time in town, I'll get you some that really fit." They walked for two hours before taking another rest. When they were near the ridge top, Gabe stopped beside a spring and refilled their canteens.

"What about those coliforms in the water you were showing your class?" she said anxiously.

"This is coming out of the rocks so it can't have much animal contamination. Being at the top of the water table keeps the human waste content down." He bent down to pull watercress from the pool and ate a handful of it with a bag of almonds. Christy tasted the greenery tentatively and was surprised to find it was good.

"How do people survive when the water was more contaminated?" she asked.

"You did pay attention. I'm totally impressed." Gabe lay back with his head on his arms. "That's an essay question. There are several answers, and they need to get all of them to get full credit. A lot of people did die from contaminated water back then. Typhoid fever was a big deal here before antibiotics and water standards. When water gets contaminated by sewage after a flood or a natural disaster, you'll notice they always talk

about the risk of disease on the news. The advantage
a long time ago was there weren't so many people to
contaminate the water, and we hadn't bred out so many
virulent strains of bacteria by slathering the earth in antibiotics. Our guts probably handle bacteria differently
with chronic exposure. You'll notice only the tourists
have to worry about Montezuma's revenge in Mexico.
The natives don't have to drink bottled water. The last
answer is that alcohol consumption may reduce how
many bacteria get through the acid in your stomach,
which may be why the apostle Paul talked about a little
wine for the stomach's sake in the Bible."

"If boiling the water kills the bacteria, then how can
bacteria live in geysers?" she asked.

"Those bacteria are really different. They don't survive out of their environment, which excludes living in
people. The ones from the vents at the bottom of the ocean
are chemosynthetic. They can make everything they need
from the elements in the water. They don't have any light
to power the chemical reactions because that deep in the
ocean there isn't any light. It's like watching a part of
the creation to see them." He sat back and took out his
compass, noting their position in a notebook.

"Do you know where we are?" Christy asked anxiously.

"I do, but I'll bet Divilbiss and his people don't.
There's no paper trail up here." He looked at Christy.
"I want you to start thinking about where that compound
is. I have a friend in Navy Intelligence, and if we can
figure out where it is, he'll help us get them. How fast
were you driving when you left?"

"It was country roads so I couldn't do more than
forty or fifty." Christy shuddered. "It was 7:30 P.M.
when we got in the car. I remember seeing the time on
the dashboard. We drove for an hour before we got to
a state highway."

"Was there a moon that night?"

Christy closed her eyes and tried to remember. She remembered turning off the headlights so they could look down at Chuck's house. The moon had been a bright beacon in the front window. She had turned the car to face it when they parked. While driving, the moon had been on her left.

"It was on my left."

"You were driving south then," Gabe told her. "The sun and moon rise in the east and set in the west. If it was on your left, the east was to your left. Did it stay there when you were driving toward the interstate?"

"Sometimes," Christy said slowly. "Sometimes it was on my left and sometimes it was almost in front of me."

"So you were forty or fifty miles north of the state highway. We'll look at a map tonight and see if we can figure which state highway. How fast were you driving on the state road?"

"The speed limit was fifty, and Chuck told me not to speed because he was afraid they might have paid off the local police. It was 9:30 P.M. when we made it to the interstate, but we detoured to Chuck's house. That took about twenty minutes because we parked above it to see if anyone was there."

"So the state road was forty miles from the interstate, and you got on before Knoxville. There aren't too many exits there because of crossing the river. Did you drive across the Clinch River, Christy? It's a long bridge and you can see smokestacks on your left even at night."

She shook her head. "I don't remember seeing a river."

"That's a big start," he reassured her. "Keep thinking. These people have money, but we've got God on our side."

They cataloged the plants along the ridge for the duration of the afternoon and had no human contact. Late in the afternoon, Gabe led the way down the windward side of the ridge to a lake. They had to wade in hip-deep water to reach the inlet where he planned to make camp. Sheer cliffs rose up behind them on three sides and offered numerous recesses where they could hide. "The only way in is the water," Gabe said. "Let's see if we can catch some supper."

Christy had never liked fish, but the smell of mountain trout frying persuaded her to try it. She realized she was ravenous from the arduous day and ate two fish along with a curious salad Gabe gathered in the woods. With no carbohydrate intake, his blood sugar was under 100 when he tested an hour later. He smiled triumphantly as he showed her the result.

"That's a message."

"This is how we would have lived two hundred years ago," she said as she moved close beside him. "I never would have imagined it would be like this. It's kind of wonderful.""

"Yes, it is," he agreed. "People drive past this country and see it as so much timber never knowing this was the garden of Eden. This was the way God meant us to live and the way we should have used food. The downside would have been that you and I probably couldn't have been together then. I would have been on the wrong side of the fort."

"I don't know and you don't either," she said. "I believe in soul mates. I would have seen you and known you were the one. I know you're the one, Gabriel. I don't think skin color or which side of the fort we were on would've made a difference. We would have run away together and lived up here." Her breath caressed his skin as she slid her hands down the front of his shirt and then under it.

"We might or should wait until it's a little darker," he said reluctantly.

"I don't want to wait." She moved to straddle his legs and pressed her body against his. She kissed him and continued kissing his neck and then his shoulders as she pulled off his fatigue jacket. It didn't take long for Christy to make Gabe forget his hesitation. It was only hard to stop long enough to take cover. They moved into a crevice where they couldn't be seen from the lake and spread out a sleeping bag. They made love while the stars rose over them and the fireflies twinkled like Christmas lights.

"I could sleep now," Christy murmured against Gabe's chest. "Just like this all night." Gabe kissed her hair and sighed.

"I wish I could let you, but we have to be ready to move." He held her face in his hands. "God must have brought us together because you know my heart when no one else ever has. Maybe He does make a perfect mate for everyone." He kissed her and sat up slowly still holding her. He was surprised to see she was wearing his dog tags. "Where did you find these?"

"On the mirror in your bedroom. I needed to have a part of you with me all the time."

"You have every part of me," he said. "Let's go for a swim."

The water was very cold, but Christy was able to ignore the temperature at first because she had never seen Gabriel swim in open water. She stayed near the shore a long time watching him and trying to imitate some of the strokes he executed. He thought nothing of swimming well away from the shore where the lake was very deep. He scared her when he dove under the water to swim back without the need to come up for air. He surfaced next to her, laughing and shaking water on her.

"Come under with me."

"I can't hold my breath that long," Christy protested. "You were underwater for a long time. How long can you hold your breath?"

"About three minutes. It's a Seal requirement. The UDT divers had to swim without tanks back in World

War II. They set a high standard to follow." He took her hand. "I'll hold onto you. Come on. Take three deep breaths and hold the last one. Squeeze my hand when you're ready to come up." She still hesitated until he put his fingers over the dog tags. "You're wearing the magic amulet for breath holding. Come with me. Keep your eyes open and look around."

She took the three deep breaths and then went under the water very conscious of her full lungs. Gabe was a very strong swimmer and pulled her along with him until she began to relax and look at the life in the lake. The water was remarkably clear. When she had to breathe, she squeezed his hand and was propelled to the surface rapidly.

"Tread water with me," he told her. "Put your hands on my arms. You don't really need anything but your legs to tread water."

"You don't." She held his arms and realized they were swimming in a circle in the middle of the lake. "It's a really long way to shore."

"This is not a long way. Ten miles is a long way. What did you think of the landscape?"

"It's like another planet," she said as she forgot to think about treading water. "Is that what the ocean is like?"

"It's even better. Someday I'll show it to you. This is Fontana Lake. TVA made it when they dammed up the Little Tennessee River. It's 580 feet deep. If we had diving gear, I could show you an underwater town."

"An underwater town?" Christy echoed.

"The town of Fontana was in the way of progress. Therefore the town was bulldozed by several million gallons of water. Every five years they drain the lake to inspect the dam, and you can see the town coming up out of its watery grave."

"Can we see it if we look under now?" Christy asked, fascinated.

"See," Gabe said. "You forgot to think about treading water or being away from shore, didn't you?" She smiled.

"You're a terrific distraction, and I have my peripheral vision. You just make me forget to use it."

"Take your breaths, and we'll go back."

He pulled her back to the shore as if she were insignificantly light, and the journey to shore wasn't nearly as threatening to Christy as the journey out had been. She would have enjoyed it if she hadn't been so cold. While she was catching her breath, Gabe realized she was shivering uncontrollably. He climbed out immediately and lifted her from the water. He wrapped a sleeping bag around her and held her against his body as if she were his child.

"I'm sorry, Christy. I didn't think about the water temperature. I had to learn to swim in such cold water that this just doesn't seem cold to me. I've had to dive in the Arctic Circle, and I remember having to keep my teeth clenched to keep from losing my mouthpiece."

"You're a frogman," she said through her chattering teeth. "I never understood that analogy until now. So if I kiss you, do you turn into a prince or stay a frogman?"

"Bad question," he said seriously. "Do you really want the answer?"

"I already know the answer," she said as she rested her head on his shoulder. "You're my prince." She sighed and kissed his neck as the warmth of his body made her warm.

"You're right, Christy." His eyes mesmerized her in the gathering darkness. "Nothing else would have mattered even two hundred years ago. I would have just carried you off." He felt her kiss his shoulder in response, and he held her close until she fell asleep in his arms. Holding her made him feel safe from all the years he had been alone. For that reason, it was hard for him to put her down even when she was asleep. The moon was high above them when he secured their camp. He tested his blood sugar and felt a rush when it was 88.

He lay down beside Christy to say prayers for both of them. He was still anguished because of Darla and Job, but during their long morning hike he had convinced himself that he couldn't have foreseen or prevented what had happened to them. The threat to Christy was much different than his previous experiences with evil. He prayed to have a better intuition about what else they might face.

CHAPTER 16

Gabe was awake before dawn and did early morning reconnaissance before awakening his wife.

"Good morning, Mrs. Killian," he whispered in her ear. "It's time to wake up." She winced as she rolled over to kiss him.

"Until yesterday I had the delusion of being in good shape. It's a downer when your thirty-something husband can run your shapely fanny into the ground."

"You did great. I'm feeling it, too, but I'm beating Bodine in the blood sugar department. Maybe we need to live up here forever." He moved to examine her leg and felt relieved when he didn't see any redness. "After we climb out of here, we'll do some stretching exercises and work the stiffness out."

"Climb out?" Christy's voice was dubious. "These rocks go straight up."

"Sure do, but it's an easy climb." His confidence was not contagious.

"Let's stay here and catch fish and swim again," she pleaded. "No one can find us here."

"I wish I could let you keep believing that, Christy, but if these people are rich enough to do what they've done, they could use satellite tracking to find us. Our greatest safety is not staying in one place long enough to confirm where we are. And, today is Tuesday. I have class tomorrow."

"Okay," she conceded. "I'm ready to be tortured again as long as I know you aren't getting some sort of sadistic paramilitary jolly out of watching me beg for mercy."

"Actually I was hoping to get several more jollies before you figured me out." He kissed her and stood with his hand extended to help her.

They ate dried fruit and another bag of almonds before Gabe started lesson one in the art of rock climbing. They did climb out of the inlet, but Christy was sure they succeeded only because Gabe was strong enough to pull her up the rock face. Her shoulders ached for two hours after they started walking. She kept her mouth shut and kept walking even when every muscle and bone in her body was protesting. She had to pray for the strength not to complain. She collapsed beside the spring where Gabe stopped to eat lunch.

"I admit it. I'm a cream puff. I'm a standard overfed poorly-muscled American girl." He laughed and handed her the canteen.

"No. I dated some of those girls. You're different. I've never met a girl who could throw inner tubes the way you do." She drank the water and then lay back.

"You're the most romantic man in America, Gabriel."

He tossed her a package of homemade granola and dried apricots. "Remember you've got to share that, Mrs. Killian."

"You can come and get it if you want it back," she challenged him. "Did you find your map?"

He delved into his backpack and pulled out a book of road maps from Tennessee, Kentucky, and North Carolina. When he found the page of interstates, he moved to sit beside her and indicated the thin red line of I-40. This is the stretch before the river. There are three exits, and I figure Oak Ridge is the most likely. This is state highway 321, and it runs north to the Tennessee state line. There's a lot of sparsely populated territory there."

"It was after the Oak Ridge exit," she said as the memory returned in a rush. "The signs pointed west to Oak Ridge and east to Knoxville. It was this exit. That was the interstate exit for Tucker, too."

"This is the Campbell state highway then. It's the only state highway within forty minutes." He marked the distance with his fingers. "Right here maybe. Did you see any landmarks, Christy? Like water towers or factory lights. Even strange road signs?"

She closed her eyes and thought of the dark highway. "There was a water tower. It was painted orange and had a Halloween pumpkin face on it. It was on the left-hand side of the road just before we got to the interstate."

"That definitely qualifies as a landmark." He took out his notebook and added to it. "Tomorrow we're going to get a topographical map and figure out where Divilbiss central is." He extended his hand requesting some of the food, and Christy tucked it into her shirt.

"Find your own food, Rambo."

"No problem." He pinned her with one arm and extracted the bags from her clothes. She was still laughing when a branch cracked just below them. Gabe was on his feet in an instant with his gun drawn. He snatched Christy off the ground and dragged her into the rocks.

Christy's heart was pounding for the first few minutes, but then as the time passed without further sounds she began to wonder if Gabe had hallucinated or at least overreacted. As she watched, he put a silencer on his handgun. He pressed his finger to his lips and left her behind the rocks. Then, he seemed to disappear right before her eyes.

The heart pounding resumed because she felt very vulnerable despite her hiding place. She felt light headed from breathing fast and sat back with her head on her arms. The click beside her sounded like thunder, and she whirled so quickly that she fell back as a bullet struck the rocks beside her. She looked into a stranger's face and knew she was going to die.

"Don't move," the man said. "I get paid whether you're alive or dead."

There was a whisper just beside her, and the man fell back, tumbling down the rocks. Christy scrambled to her feet and started running in sheer terror. She had run fifty yards when Gabe caught her, but for several moments she didn't recognize him. She fought his grasp until they both fell.

"It's okay, Christy." He was breathing as hard as she was, but his hands weren't sweating, and his heartbeat seemed much slower than hers was. "I got them. They're dead."

She sobbed with the effort of breathing and clung to Gabe even when he lifted her to her feet. Her legs were shaking so hard she felt like they weren't going to hold her weight. Gabe kept her on her feet until he eased her down to sit near the spring again. He confiscated the guns from the fallen men and methodically searched both bodies before dragging them to lie side by side. He covered the bodies with a silver colored tarp. Then he took out the radio and flipped up the antenna.

"Hawkeye, this is Windrunner." There was a short static filled pause.

"Go ahead, Windrunner."

"I've got some specimens you might be interested in. Can you get these coordinates?"

"That's a roger, Windrunner. Can you mark the specimens?"

"They'll be waiting for you. Pick us up at the drop off at five in the morning. Windrunner out." He closed the radio and dropped to one knee to repack his bag. "Let's go, Christy. It won't seem so bad when you don't have to look at them."

They walked out of the mountains without any pretense of surveying. It took the rest of the day to reach Deep Creek, and Gabe made their camp in another rock face well off the beaten path. He dug into his pack to produced a package of jerky to eat with fern fronds and wild mushrooms, but Christy had no appetite for it. She drank her portion of the water and lay down on her sleeping bag as the moon began rising. Gabe sat down beside her and caressed her hair gently.

"I'm sorry, Christy. I wish it didn't have to be this way."

"It's my fault," she murmured. "You're having to do this because of me. I wish it were over. I keep praying it will be over." He put down his gun and pulled her into his lap to hold her tightly.

"It's a test of our faith, Christy. Think about it that way, and it will be easier. I don't think God tests someone unless He believes they're strong enough to pass the test and to grow from taking it. Together we're going to be strong enough." He kissed her hair. "I know we're going to get out of this so don't be afraid. God always follows people who wander in the wilderness."

His words and his eyes convinced her. She managed to relax in his arms because he made her feel safe when the idea of safety defied logic. She slept while Gabe held her and kept watch. He couldn't have slept that night. How close they had come to disaster was holding his mind captive. He had believed he could elude their pursuers. That night he had to accept that it was very different from his past experiences to be the prey. He began to brace himself for the real possibility that he might have to leave the place he called home.

He awakened Christy at sunrise and led her down territory they had crossed days earlier. Christy didn't recognize any of it.

They climbed down to the bulletproof car at five o'clock in the morning. Christy could tell Gabe was as tired as she was. She felt much calmer after her sleep, but she slid across the backseat of the FBI car and closed her eyes to relish the moments of relative protection.

"Did you find what I left you?" Gabe asked.

"Yeah, and we've got positive ID on both of them. They're known paramilitary and most recently paid assassins. That was nice shooting, Killian. One bullet each right through the heart. You must have been keeping up with your craft."

"I don't believe in overstating my capabilities," Gabe replied. "Do you know how my cousin is doing?"

"Upgraded to stable and out of intensive care. He was airlifted to the regional trauma center at Mercy Hospital, but the agent there says he's talking and moving everything. He didn't see anything or at least doesn't remember seeing anything."

"Thank God," Gabe sighed. "We need to shower and get changed before class. Did you make sure my house is secure?"

"It's secure," the agent replied. "We've got five people around it now, but I think you took out the problem."

"For now," Gabe said. "After my class I want to show you the map we've put together. We've got a better idea of where Christy was held."

"Good," the agent said, but Gabe knew the word signified a lack of commitment. He sat back with his eyes closed and began formulating his fall-back plan.

There was relief in finding the house was still intact though festooned with the yellow crime scene tapes. Gabe carried in both backpacks and bent to turn on the strip of lights on the floor. The windows had been covered with tin foil to prevent any telltale shadows or thermal images from being seen outside.

"Watch your step, Christy," Gabe said. "It's dark in here." He led her through the house to the bathroom and closed the door behind them. "Let's get a shower and put the fatigues in the wash. Then we'll get some real food."

"I'm glad you said that. I felt guilty about my unhealthy craving for chocolate." She stripped off her jacket, hat, and pants hurriedly and turned on the hot water. Gabe moved close behind her and pulled her back against his body.

"I'm only craving you," he said. She closed her eyes and relaxed against him as he removed the rest of her clothes. His hands seemed to touch every part of her before he pulled her into the shower with him. The hot water was soothing, but it was Gabe who washed away her fears as he held her. They stayed under the water a long time.

"You keep saving my life," she said as she passed him a towel and then paused to dry his back. "How can this be a reciprocal relationship when you're the main caretaker."

"When we get settled, I'll let you take over." He pulled on a clean pair of boxers and gave her the bathrobe hanging behind the door. "I'll meet you in the bedroom. I can't promise to behave. I will promise to be good."

She smiled when she didn't really feel like smiling and followed him to the dark bedroom. Gabe found her new clothes by touch and gave her jeans and an embroidered denim shirt.

"You get to be gorgeous today. Don't make me jealous."

"You don't have any reason to worry, Gabriel. I'm helplessly in love with you. On the other hand, I saw how some of the girls in your class were looking at you. Just make sure they see your wedding ring."

"I didn't notice because you were getting all my attention." He kissed her bare shoulder and held her for another reassuring moment. He located dress slacks and an earth tone shirt while she dressed. Christy started the laundry and breakfast to give Gabe time to prepare for his classes. They had just enough time to eat before they needed to depart for the college.

Christy had intended to listen to the lecture and the discussion of the students' essays, but she was exhausted. At the end of the lecture, her head was resting on her folded arms. She slept through the remainder of the class. As he prepared to dismiss the class, Gabe was taking questions from his students. Josh Turney raised his hand.

"Dr. Killian, this is a little off the subject, but some of us were noticing you have a new piece of jewelry, and we were wondering about it."

Gabe held up his left hand. "I presume you mean this piece of jewelry, Mr. Turney. If I'm correct in my assumption, you can discover the significance of this type of jewelry in sociology books that discuss American marriage customs."

There were numerous whistles, catcalls, and assorted claps through the classroom. Gabe put up with the banter for several minutes and then said, "Are there any other relevant questions?"

Allan Story raised his hand, grinning as Gabe pointed to him. "Dr. Killian, we were just wondering why Mrs. Killian couldn't stay awake in class?"

"She's been studying biology, Mr. Story. We've been staying up late at night studying biology." Classroom decorum ended in laughter, and Gabe turned to erase the board as a signal that class was dismissed. His special topics class came into the room as the rest of the environmental biology class departed, and he spent two hours with them.

"I guess we've been married long enough for you to get bored," he whispered in Christy's ear as he awakened her.

"I need about eighteen hours of uninterrupted sleep," she murmured. "I really wanted to listen but the sleep center in my brain overrode everything else."

"That's not a bad excuse, and I'm a real hard case about excuses." He led her to his office and flipped on his laptop to call up an internet search engine. Within minutes, a detailed map of Tennessee appeared on the screen. Gabe enlarged the area several times and then printed both the topography and the roads. Then he called up a map showing how to get to Tucker College and began searching into the college's infrastructure. When he called up the Board of Directors, the name Divilbiss appeared twice.

"Well, well. It would seem Tucker might be involved. I wonder if the county records show what else the Divilbiss family owns." He began searching county by county. After two hours he hadn't found any rural properties owned by a Divilbiss.

"Dead end. They must have a corporate name." He flipped to e-mail and sent a message to Tracy Tolliver.

"Tracer, we both know paybacks are always a challenge. Before you say no, remember who took a bullet to keep your butt in one piece. I need you to get into whatever nationally-secured database it takes to find out about Carlton Divilbiss. I need to know every corporation he's involved in. His date of birth is 10/16/49. I could also use a list of every property he and his corporation claimed on their income tax. My wife and I have been threatened and shot at by people Divilbiss hired. If I don't get more help than what the feds are willing to give, you'll be getting invited to my funeral. Windrunner."

His personal e-mail was uninteresting. He closed his laptop and looked back at Christy. She was asleep again with her head on her arm. She looked like a little girl, and Gabe felt a fresh rush of rage because she was being made to suffer. He kissed her temple.

"Come on, baby. Let's go home."

CHAPTER 17

With the agents to guard them and the house secured, Gabe chose to take the risk of remaining in Cherokee another night. He transmitted his survey results and lay down beside his wife for a ten-hour nap. When he emerged to make tea the next morning, the head agent, Hawkeye, was sitting at the kitchen table pouring over his notes and the two maps.

"I was beginning to think we did all that for nothing," Gabe said.

"I want to see any leads you have," Hawkeye said, "but don't expect me to saddle my horse and take the cavalry over the hill to capture them until we have a whole lot more."

"I've always considered myself too quick on the smart comments, but I have to ask just what you are going to do now?" Gabe asked. "I know all about stretching international laws so give me a break from the rhetoric. You have every reason to believe they're holding people against their will. Satellites don't just cruise over Libya and Iraq you know."

"You're involved in this case, Killian, but don't think you have any say in what happens," Hawkeye said sharply.

"Rock on, General Custer, and we'll see who's still standing when this is over," Gabe retorted. "The two things every Native American has learned from history is don't negotiate with white men bearing peace treaties, and don't wait until dawn to attack."

"Listen, smart ass, I'm on your side," Hawkeye said. "When I started looking into this, the people at Tucker College called the local police. They accused your wife of killing Chuck Portman. I found that fascinating since I had just done a search on Portman, and there's no record of such a person ever existing. When I told them that, they backed off. You need to remember I didn't have to defend her. I could have just taken her into custody."

The agent had no way of knowing he had pushed Gabe Killian's button until he was standing toe to toe with an irate ex-Seal. Gabe had the ability to be very intimidating.

"Don't threaten me, and don't threaten her," Gabe snapped. "You know my background or you wouldn't have chosen that particular threat. I have friends in high places, too, and it might be time for me to call in my chips. If I do, you may not like the hand you get dealt."

Hawkeye picked up the map and shoved it into Gabe's hands. "Show me what you've really got, and I'll see what the satellites can get us."

Gabe showed him everything Christy had remembered and then returned to the bedroom with a cup of tea to awaken his wife. She stretched and sat up smiling.

"Okay. I'm recharged now."

"You're faster than I am. I'm still trying to work out kinks. We may just lay around until dusk and then hit the trail."

"How long will we be running like this, Gabe?"

"This isn't running," he asserted. "This is surveying. Anybody who thinks they want to follow us had better start running." He leaned against the headboard and pulled her back against his body. "If they can't get them, we'll go into the witness protection program."

"You'd lose your family and your home," Christy protested. "You've told me how much your heritage means to you, Gabriel. You can't give up all that for me."

"You became my first priority last Friday when I married you." He held her tightly. "You and I are a family now, Christy. We're going to do whatever we have to do to keep this family safe. I'm not going to argue about it so surrender now and save time." He turned her to look into his eyes. "You've made me happier in the last few days than I've ever been. I prayed to know where I should go, and I think I have my answer."

She forced herself to smile as she looked into his heart. "You told me your eagle feather means more to you than anything in the house. If we went into the witness program, you couldn't have it on the wall."

"What it stands for is what I cherish. It's about being a warrior and making the right decisions. What it stands for will always be in my heart. No one can take that away. That's just a part of being strong hearted." He kissed her. "God never asks you for more than you can give, Christy. Before I had you, having my home here was important. Now I'll be taking home with me wherever I go."

Christy was too moved to do anything more than hold onto her husband for several moments. Then she whispered, "I used to think I was in a place where it was always night. I kept waiting for the sunrise because the Bible says joy comes in the morning. You've been my sunrise."

That night, with Gabe's arms securely around her, she starting praying for God to make her a Deborah so she could stand and fight beside her husband. When they were dropped off deep inside the park that night, she didn't feel quite so afraid. Leaving her fear behind her allowed her to live each day as it came and not worry about the morrow.

Gabe brought a sketch pad and a set of acrylic pastels he had used to make biological drawings. Christy used those to make drawings of every sunset. When it was too dark to draw, Gabe taught her more martial arts moves and how to use his handgun. She was surprised to learn he had both handguns from their attackers.

"Why did you keep them?"

"To increase our arsenal," Gabe said. He was silent for a moment and then said, "I probably should give them to Hawkeye so he can check the ballistics on the bullet that killed Darla, but it had to be a sniper's rifle and not a handgun. I also wanted to be able to prove we've been fired on. Once the evidence is out of our hands, we can't get it back." Reality returned in a rush.

"You're saying you could get in trouble for shooting them."

"No. I'm saying I'm going to make sure I don't get in trouble for shooting them. I didn't have to think about that when I was a Seal. That was a battlefield situation, and if somebody else has a gun, they're a target. It can't be that way here." He lifted her chin and looked into her eyes. "I know what I'm doing, Christy. Don't worry."

She chose to believe he was in control because the belief allowed her to sleep at night.

They stopped at a tiny town on the edge of the park Sunday morning and replenished their supplies. Gabe paid in cash, and no one paid them any attention. Feeling safe from pursuit, they attended the little church in the town. They stayed in the back and left hurriedly at the end of the service. They had just reentered the park when a ranger called out to them.

"Are you guys with a group? You're off the usual trail."

Gabe produced his Park Service ID. "We're field biologists doing survey work." The ranger examined the card and returned it.

"You need to be careful. There was a murder in the park yesterday. Two hikers alone over near Cherokee were shot and killed."

Christy's hands tightened on her backpack straps. "Why? Was it a robbery?"

"They were stalked and shot execution style," the ranger said grimly. "We don't know why yet. You might want to stay near the usual campgrounds."

"We're almost finished," Gabe said. "Thanks for the warning. You never know what kind of nuts you'll find even in the park."

"Pass the word along." The ranger tipped his hat to them and turned his horse back toward the trail. Christy moved close to Gabe and put her damp hand on his arm.

"They were after us, Gabe."

"You don't know that," he said tersely. "Let's go."

They were headed back toward Cherokee, but Gabe took them high into the mountains that day. They made their camp beside a lake in another isolated inlet. Christy went swimming to cool off because it had been a hot, humid day for the mountains. Gabe sat on the bank with his fishing pole staring out over the water. When Christy climbed out, he had caught four fish and had his line cast a fifth time.

"I think we probably have enough supper." She pulled on clean underwear and a tee shirt. "You're thinking about those people."

"I'm wondering how to end this," he said as he pulled in his line. "We can stay out of their way, but I don't like to think of innocent people dying in my place. I sent my buddy in Naval Intelligence an e-mail asking him to help us. He has access to every database in the United States. Carlton Divilbiss is on the Board of Directors at Tucker so he's probably using the school to collect victims. I think someone is going to have to go into the compound and get evidence because the federal people are afraid of ever having another Waco scenario. I'm beginning to think the Seals are much better trained than federal operatives. Compared to what we had to do, this kind of reconnaissance is pretty tame. My idea of risk is being dropped into Sadaam Hussein's back yard. Maybe Tracer and I can do what needs to be done." She was in his lap almost immediately and held his face in her hands.

"I don't want you to take the risk, Gabriel. I don't want to take any risk of losing you. We've only been together a few days, but already I feel like we're the only man and woman on earth—like we're Adam and Eve. It's a wonderful feeling. I love you so much. Don't make me give you up. I couldn't stand losing you."

Gabe had enjoyed danger and risk, but the promise of one last mission couldn't compete with the expression on Christy's face. Any doubts he had had about the depths of her feelings had long since faded. The need to punish anyone connected with Divilbiss was being tempered by his personal experience with the price of violence.

"I'm not going to let anything come between us," he said soothingly. "I promise I won't take any risks. I won't do anything you ask me not to do."

"Please don't ever leave me," she begged him. "I'd rather be dead than feel how I felt when I didn't have you." She clung to him and kissed him with desperate passion. She pushed him back on the bank with her hands holding her body tightly against his body. When she stopped trembling, Gabe pulled her into the lake again, but he knew he wasn't really able to make her forget her fear that night. She hid it from him, but he was all too aware of her feelings. She didn't talk about them until after they had finished eating.

"Would you be all right if we had to go into the witness program, Gabriel?"

"I really would," he said. "I found the perfect passage in the Bible. It ought to be the witness protection motto. It's where Ruth is telling Naomi she wanted to come with her to her own country. 'Whither thou goest, I will go and whither thou lodgest, I will lodge. Thy people will be my people and thy God, my God. Whither thou diest, I will die and there will I be buried. The Lord do so to me and more also if ought but death part me and thee.' That's how marriage is supposed to be." He took her hands and held them both.

"Maybe we won't have to leave Cherokee, Christy, but I'll be fine if we do for however long it takes to get Divilbiss. I hope it isn't forever; but even if I knew it would be, I'd rather go away than think about people dying in my place. One of the most revered men from the time of removal was a man named Tsali. When my people were fighting to stay here, he gave his life to keep the army from looking for all the others. Courage is realizing what you want may not be the best thing for everyone else." He paused.

"I need to finish my survey. If we keep up this pace, I can finish it this week. I'd also like to finish my class if I can. There's no one else to teach it, and those students are depending on me. Then we're going to do what's best for this family." She looked relieved and picked up her sketch pad.

"I guess we'll be spending the next few weeks in the garden of Eden, and I can't say I'm sorry. I'll make drawings and paint some memories for us while we're away. I've also got a few other ways to spend our time when we're home for you to teach class."

"And those are?" Gabe asked.

"Oh, I was thinking about having you put on your uniform. You know the white one." Her eyes teased him as she smiled. "Then I can either draw your picture wearing it, or alternatively I can take it off of you one piece at a time."

"Do I get to choose?" he asked. Christy pointed to his notebook.

"Do your homework, and I'll draw the sunset. And yes. You get to choose."

"I think you should know I'm putting that idea on the top of my agenda for when we get home. That's a big step for me because I'm totally obsessive compulsive about the condition of my uniform. This is major proof of where you rank." He picked up his notebook and then said, "You know that movie is about Navy pilots and not Navy divers, don't you?"

"I know," Christy said. "I'm afraid of heights. I love the water." She looked over her sketch pad and saw he was smiling. Then she worked on her drawing, which wasn't of the sunset. While Gabe was occupied with his report, Christy was perfecting a drawing of her husband and how he might have looked in a world two hundred years earlier. She was so intent that she didn't notice he had moved behind her and was looking down at her work.

"If that's me, I'm tremendously flattered," he said. "You know my hair was that long pre-Navy."

"It's you. Job gave me a guided tour of your photo albums," she admitted. "So why didn't you grow your hair long again when you got out?"

He spread out their sleeping bags side by side before answering. "This is long compared to nine years of crew cuts." He sat down beside her and caressed her hair. "I really like your hair, so do me a favor and don't ever cut it. I'll bet you didn't know red has always been my favorite color." He pulled her back to lean against him and watched her draw until the light faded to stars. Then Christy lay down looking up at the constellations with her head on his arm.

"I'll bet you know every constellation," she said.

"Not all of them, but I can find most of them. You know they have different names to the Cherokee. When

I was a kid, Qualla Boundary wasn't quite as populated, especially in the spring and late fall.

You could lay out in Jonah's back yard and watch the stars come out. You know the signs of the Zodiac are all constellations, and they rotate around the north pole. It takes fifty-two years for them to make a complete revolution, and yet the Egyptians and the Mayans knew that. They built their temples that way by adding a layer or building a new one every fifty-two years. They've done DNA probes on the Mayas in the Yucatan, and they're genetically similar to the Chinese. I used to think about getting into anthropology and archeology to research the history of our tribe. There's so much culture that's been lost. I do want our children to know about being Cherokee."

"They will. We don't have to go light years away from here, and maybe we won't have to stay away. Let's just pray for God to show us the way we should go." She said the prayer with her eyes on the heavens. As she said, "Amen," a meteor streaked toward the earth and disappeared just above the trees. Gabe's hand tightened on her shoulder telling her he had also seen it.

CHAPTER 18

Gabe and Christy radioed the federal agent on Tuesday night and were picked up on the road to Maggie Valley at 5 A.M. on Wednesday. The agent was accompanied by two partners and scarcely gave them time to settle themselves in the van before he related the events of the week.

"Your enemies have been very busy. Three couples hiking in the park were killed this week. All of them were couples with dark-haired men and red-headed women. The agency is making your case a priority now because there's talk the Park Service might close the park down until the perpetrators are caught. The agency doesn't want to contemplate what would happen if the park were closed during peak tourist season. The hotels and resorts would probably burn us in effigy."

"Six bodies too late," Gabe thought. He might have voiced the thought except for Christy's hand squeezing his arm. He realized she was aware of his hostile thoughts when he looked at her.

"Did you find the compound?" Christy asked.

"Maybe," the agent responded. "We've had the satellites covering a two hundred square mile area around the exit and state roads you indicated. There are six enclosures bound in chain-length fence but only one has barbed wire on top of it. I need you to look at the photos and see if we've found the right place. For now, we've code named it, *blood farm*."

"Are there people there?" Christy asked, shuddering.

"Yes," the agent replied. "More than a few so we need to be as sure as we can be that we're looking at the right place. We thought you could look at the pictures while your husband was teaching his class."

"No," Gabe said adamantly. "Christy had to run for her life to escape that compound and watch the man who helped her die. When she has to relive it, I'm going to be with her. We'll do it this afternoon." Hawkeye shot a glance at Gabe and shrugged.

"This afternoon will be fine, Dr. Killian. Try not to be so defensive. We're on your side."

"Forgive me if I withhold my final judgment." Gabe pulled Christy close beside him and closed his eyes for the duration of the ride. He felt paranoid and too angry to be rational when they reached his house, so he focused on his class. He showered hurriedly and went to his computer to prepare an essay exam for his class. He printed seventeen copies and then took out six sealed soil samples he had collected. Christy came bearing tea, cheese, and fruit.

"I know Mr. Bodine said no breakfast, but you're losing weight. Please eat." She ran her hands over his muscular shoulders. "I think you've already lost ten of the fifteen pounds he thought you should lose. He should be pleased."

"I'm happy even if he isn't. I'm back down to 178. That's the best weight I've had since I started graduate school. I feel like I'm doing all we can do to treat the diabetes right now. I've passed being freaked out, and I'm ready to learn more. I'm going to try and download more educational materials to take with us."

"What made you feel more at ease?" she asked.

"Seeing I can control the blood sugars. I thought I could keep myself from getting diabetes. When it happened despite everything I did for three years, I felt like I was at the mercy of it. Bodine made me understand. This happened because of all the years that I didn't know how to protect my pancreas. I used to love to drink soda. When I was in the Navy, I could kill a six pack of soda by myself every day. The only reason my weight stayed down was because I was moving eighteen hours a day. I have a feeling that insulin is like a bank account in your pancreas. You're born with enough to last all your life unless you spend it all on junk food and soda when you're young.

"When we have kids, we're going to teach them not to eat sugar and fat. If I have to have deal with diabetes so our kids won't, that's a small price to pay. Maybe they'll have less risk anyway because I put some new genes into the family pool. Bodine said the tendency to have diabetes definitely runs in families as well as ethnic populations. Is there any diabetes in your family?"

"Not that I know. Most of the great aunts and uncles died of old age. My mother's parents were killed in accidents, too. Her father was in a factory explosion. Her mother died in a car accident. My father's father died in the Korean War. My grandmother died from a blood clot after she broke her hip, but she was eighty years old. I don't know of anyone with diabetes or heart disease, but my father's family was English. Mr. Bodine said people of English descent are more at risk, just like African Americans and Native Americans are."

"If your family didn't get it, maybe they had some sort of genetic protection. With that, diet and exercise, maybe we can keep our kids from having it at all." His attitude reaffirmed that he was ready to fight against diabetes and carried the idea that it was something they could defeat.

"I don't think I could have gotten my head straight so quickly without you, Christy. I have a reason not to let the emotions bog me down because I want to have a family with you. I don't expect you to manage my disease, but it's easier to fight a battle when someone you trust is backing you up."

The words made her happy. She knew they were growing closer every day despite the adversity she had brought into Gabriel's life. She kissed him for several minutes, almost letting herself forget they had other things to accomplish.

"Maybe you'd better stop before I forget about my class," Gabe said reluctantly. "I don't think my department chairman would excuse my absence even if I had a note from my wife." He kissed her neck. "Get dressed."

Christy spent the day drawing while the class analyzed soil samples and then placed them in an incubator to see what seeds would germinate. The lab was followed by the examination that was a series of essay questions. It took the students almost two hours to complete them. When that class departed, four students doing Gabe's independent study course arrived and spent the remainder of the day with him. Gabe was packing his briefcase when Jonah came into the room and walked up to his desk. It was obvious that Gabe was very glad to see his uncle and equally obvious that Jonah didn't blame them for his son's injury.

"I've been worried, but I see God answered my prayers. You're looking very well." He smiled at Christy. "You've been good for him."

"How's Job?" Gabe asked.

"He's home. I wish you could see him. He's taking Darla's death very hard. He doesn't blame you, Gabe.

He knows he and Darla shouldn't have been alone together at your house. You couldn't have prevented what happened. You've done well staying out of harm's way and taking care of your bride."

"We may have to leave here, Jonah," Gabe said reluctantly.

"I had thought you might." Jonah took two silver crosses from his pocket and put them in Gabe's hand. "These are your wedding presents from Reba and me. If you do have to leave, Gabe, think of Florida. The Seminole and Cherokee people share a similar heritage and similar customs. You have always loved the sea, and they say there is need for field biologists to study the fresh water springs. On the Seminole reservation you could still work to better a Native American people."

Gabe embraced his uncle for a long moment and then seemed to make a great effort to speak without emotion.

"If we do have to go, they may tell you that we're dead." His voice broke, and he hesitated before saying, "I'll get word to you some way and let you know we're all right."

"You've made the right choices, Gabe," Jonah said gently. "Now, I'm also sure that Christy is the one God meant for you to marry. Pray with her every day, and God will bless your marriage." He turned to Christy and put his hands on her shoulders. "And you are now my daughter like Gabe is my son. You should pray with your husband and children every day. I know you will be a virtuous wife and mother." He kissed her cheek and walked away leaving Christy to see the sadness Gabe couldn't hide. She held onto her husband's arm as they walked out to join the federal agents.

Instead of being taken home, they were taken to a multimedia room on campus and shown the satellite photographs. Gabe was sure the agents would attempt to deceive Christy to test her credibility as a witness.

He was correct in his assumption. The agents showed them numerous photographs of fenced enclosures, and Christy shook her head at each of the first twenty. Gabe knew when they had the real blood farm on the screen because she started trembling.

"That's it," she said, her voice quavering.

"You're sure?" the agent asked.

"I'm sure." She pointed to a low flat building. "That's where they take the blood. That's where we lived." The agent switched off the projector.

"It's just outside of Olive Springs, Tennessee. That's about forty miles from Tucker College. Divilbiss has a mansion and outbuildings on the other side of the property. It won't be an easy place to enter."

Gabe walked over to the projector and flipped the switch. As the image reappeared, he pointed to a grayish line.

"Is this a river running through it?" He scanned the agent's face to obtain his answer. "There won't be any problem doing reconnaissance if you think *under* instead of *over*. What kind of evidence are you going after?"

"Something that will get us a formal warrant to search the place. I'd like to think there are bodies buried in the compound."

"I'll bet they're too smart to have the evidence there," Gabe said. He took the topographical map out of his briefcase and circled the position of the compound. He tapped on a nearby depression with his pen.

"Is this an abandoned quarry? It looks to be maybe two miles from the compound. That kind of lake is deep. You can hide all sorts of dead bodies in a quarry lake. Why don't you have a look?" Hawkeye's face told Gabe he was about to get another excuse. He hoped he was wrong because his fuse was too short to hear any more excuses.

There was a knock at the door that fortuitously interrupted the impending confrontation. The two agents reached for their guns before a female voice called, "It's Janie, Dr. Killian. I have a package for you. It's from Commander Tolliver at Annapolis."

Gabe went to the door but opened it hesitantly until he could ascertain that the departmental secretary was alone. He had wondered how to make certain the package was safe to open. When he saw the package was held by his comrade, security became a moot point. The two former Seals embraced as they greeted each other.

"Tracer, you're a lifesaver," Gabe said.

"Windrunner, teachers aren't supposed to get into this kind of trouble." Tracy Tolliver surveyed the two agents and then smiled broadly on seeing Christy. "This must be your bride. How'd you get a girl this pretty to settle for your ugly mug?"

"Christy," Gabe said, "this is Commander Tracy Tolliver. Forgive his incredible lack of manners. I tried to teach him how to behave in public, but it would take an act of God. Tracy, this is my wife, Christy."

Tracy grinned as he extended his hand to Christy. "It's good to meet you, Mrs. Killian. I'll tell you the whole dirty truth about your husband later." He tossed the package to Gabe.

"Ask and it shall be given. Carlton Divilbiss is a real piece of excrement, if you get my drift. He's into every crime that can be committed in the United States including drug running and money laundering. He's the proud owner of nineteen bogus corporations, and there's a list of the land he's claiming behind the second page."

"Why couldn't we get this kind of intelligence work when we were getting shot at?" Gabe opened the package hurriedly and flipped to the land document. "Olive Branch Farm. A nice, neat two-hundred acre plantation." Gabe looked at Tracy. "The investigation has been slow to get started. Did you bring any diving gear? There's a quarry we need to check out."

"Have wet suit, will travel," Tracy assured him.

CHAPTER 19

They were taken to Gabe's house, and Christy cooked a big meal for the five men while Gabe and Tracy talked and planned the dive at the quarry. The thought of Gabe risking himself terrified her. She stood at the kitchen sink and prayed, "I need to be Deborah, God. I really need to be Deborah."

She set the table and served the food, forcing herself to eat it while she thought of the three couples who had died. Gabe was going only to look for evidence, and she knew he needed to do it to prevent more deaths. Still, she couldn't stop worrying after the dishes were done and the laundry was folded. An agent kept watch in the kitchen while she worked, and she tried to make conversation.

"Why did you put tin foil over the windows?"

"You can't read thermal images through it," the unknown agent said tersely.

"What are thermal images?" she asked not knowing how disconcerting knowledge could be.

"There are gun sites that let you target a warm body," the agent said. "You can be killed by a gunman who never sees your face."

It was a moment when the fear overpowered her, and Christy went to the bedroom and lay down to pray herself to sleep. It was no easy task. The last time she looked at the clock, it read midnight.

A sound startled Christy from sleep, and she sat up with her heart racing.

"Gabriel?"

"It's me," she heard him say from the closet.

"What time is it?" Christy asked as she tried to exhale her fright.

"It's about one o'clock. Time for you to make good on your promise," he said. She was bewildered until he appeared from the closet wearing his dress white uniform. Christy couldn't keep from smiling because he had again pushed her fears aside.

"You look great," she said as she crossed the room. "You look whole lots better than the guy in the movie."

"I doubt that. Richard Gere was in that movie." She looked up into his eyes and then stood on tiptoe to kiss him.

"Like you said about Joannie. Not to me, Gabriel. No one could ever look as good as you look to me." He put his hat on her head and picked her up. She put her arms around his neck still smiling. "You've seen the movie."

He couldn't suppress his own smile as he carried her to the bed and sat down beside her.

"I saw the movie. I'm here seeking equality for Navy divers everywhere. I've already had a huge rush because my uniform still fits almost five years after discharge. It's not even tight."

Christy pushed him down and leaned over him with her hair all around them. "Don't think I'm not appreciating how well it fits you. I promise to wash and iron your uniform. So just relax and put yourself and your dress whites in my hands."

"I think you should put yourself in my hands," he said as he pulled her close. What followed was a school girl dream of Christy's, and her husband made it come true for her. She was almost asleep in his arms when she heard him whisper, "Someday, when all this is over, we'll have another wedding. I'll wear the dress whites for you. We can let Jonah do the ceremony and get you a real wedding dress."

"You don't have to do all that," she protested. "Our little ceremony in Asheville was wonderful."

"I want to do it for you, Christy. I want to do anything that makes you happy."

She had no trouble sleeping when he was holding her. Gabe woke her up early the next morning kissing her temple. His breath tickled her, and she smiled.

"If you say, guess who, I already know."

"Good morning, Mrs. Killian," he said as she turned to face him. "Hawkeye has made arrangements to get us to that quarry lake. I'm sure it was under the duress of knowing two Seals against one federal agent wouldn't be a fair fight, but at least we're going. We'll need to leave in about thirty minutes. Do you want to go?"

"I'll be ready in ten minutes," she replied. "You're not going anywhere without me."

She hurried to shower and change into jeans and a tee shirt. While she was braiding her hair, she tried not to watch Gabriel ready his diving gear.

"How deep is the water there, Gabe?" she asked with a racing heart.

"Probably a hundred feet or so. Not real deep by Navy standards." Gabe scanned her anxious face. "Christy, this is like a diving class for me. I was qualified in the special suits for deep water. Real deep water. I've had to go through decompression to get back to the surface."

"Like down the Cayman Wall deep water?"

"Deeper than that. Did you ever see the movie, *The Abyss*?" Gabe asked.

"That's deep." Christy's eyes widened. "OK. I guess this is a swimming pool for you. Just be careful."

He kissed her pale lips. "You pray. I'll dive."

A van came to get them and took them across the mountains into Tennessee. A helicopter picked them up outside of Pigeon Forge, and unlike the tour helicopters, it was clearly military and flew very fast and quietly across the countryside. When they were near enough to the compound for Christy to recognize the terrain, Gabe and Tracy began getting on their wet suits. Christy hadn't realized they would be stripping to the skin until Gabe directed her to look away.

"I don't want Tracy to be humiliated by the comparison," Gabe laughed.

"You don't want her to be jealous of what she could've had," Tracy jibed.

Gabe suited up first and checked both sets of tanks and two sets of goggles designed for diving in murky water. He returned to Christy's side.

"If we find what we're looking for, you won't want to see it. Don't look if we bring anything up."

"You guys ready?" Hawkeye asked.

"Get us no more than twenty feet over the water," Tracy requested. "We don't know what's under the surface, and I don't want to find out by hitting it." He and Gabe moved to opposites sides of the helicopter and climbed out on the struts as they descended over the quarry. Moments later they dropped feet first into the water and disappeared. Christy closed her hand over the silver cross Jonah had given her along with Gabriel's dog tags. Then she closed her eyes tightly and prayed.

Gabe was surprised by the impenetrable blackness of the water because quarry lakes were usually clear. Being a Seal had required him to dive into deep water at night so he was experienced in keeping his orientation. It was difficult to locate Tracy for several minutes, and finding his partner was his first goal. He couldn't proceed alone. When he found Tracy, they moved as a team toward the bottom of the lake watching their depth gages with surprise. The bottom was almost two hundred feet down, and they couldn't see it until they were almost on it. The bottom was uneven and studded with junked cars and abandoned appliances, constant hazards for divers. Tracy moved ahead slightly to look in some of the cars, but Gabe stayed along the deep mud always keeping Tracy in sight.

After some fifteen minutes of searching, he was rewarded by finding an arm. When he followed the curiously preserved limb, he quickly found himself in a gruesome underwater cemetery. The rocks were draped with bodies in various states of decomposition. He swam to where Tracy was and summoned his partner. Tracy returned with him to the graveyard and froze for a moment as he absorbed the scene. When he recovered his composure, Tracy unfolded a net to wrap the first body. While they were wrapping it, they found treasure.

Gabe and Tracy came to the surface together and waved for the helicopter. The thumbs up signal informed the agents that they had been successful. The helicopter began its descent while lowering a basket on a long cable. The body was loaded first and then the same winch lifted the divers. The helicopter was moving away from the quarry before Gabe and Tracy were inside. When they had secured the door, Gabe tossed a bag on the floor dumping some thirty laminated ID's.

"I'll bet some of these people have families who filed missing person reports," Gabe said. "There must be fifty bodies on the south side of the lake. Is that enough probable cause?"

The agent's response was noncommittal.

"Give me a day or two to research these IDs and get an identity on this body. We may have to recover more of them to get a federal warrant."

Gabe looked at Tracy who shook his head. They both stood and began stripping off their gear. Christy kept her face averted until they were dressed. Gabe moved to put his arms around her before she could come to him.

"I know her, Gabriel. Her name is Bernice Callahan. She disappeared just before I escaped. I saw her body the night Chuck helped me."

She was shaking in his arms, and Gabe pulled her head down on his shoulder and held her more securely.

"It could have been you, baby. Just keep remembering God spared you. None of this was your fault." She had never thought she would like being called baby, but every time Gabe said the word, she felt protected and loved. She was also sure he hadn't ever said it to another woman. She held onto him and tried to forget the sight of Bernice's body.

The helicopter ride to Sevier County was quick, but the drive back to Cherokee seemed to take forever. They didn't stop for food, and even Gabe was ready to eat when they reached his house. The agents guarding the house had ordered pizza, and the group was quick to use it as an appetizer. While Gabe was showering, Christy made spaghetti with marinara sauce for their real meal. She made Gabe a large salad. When she was cleaning up the kitchen, Gabe and Tracy had a private conversation in Job's room.

"You may be slightly over your head, Gabe," Tracy said. "Divilbiss would be looking at life without parole or the death penalty, so he's got nothing to lose by coming after you with both barrels blazing."

"I've got the big picture, Tracy. I just don't have a lot of options. They don't consider us as witnesses until they make a case. I guess they want a taped confession. I would think that underwater cemetery would be enough, but I'm just a biology teacher. What do I know about crime and punishment?"

"It impressed me. It was the most gruesome thing I've seen since 'storm.' I'll go see Rick and Jimmy at the CIA office. Maybe they can put a little pressure on these bureaucratic butt heads. In the meantime, keep your head down and take care of your bride. She's something special. Losing your peripheral vision may have been the luckiest thing that ever happened to you."

"I've been thinking that same thing," Gabe said.

Christy retreated to the bedroom as soon as the kitchen was clean and sat with the sketch pad in her lap remembering all the people. She was listing them when Gabe came to see about her. He closed the door behind him and sat down on the bed beside her to test his blood sugar. It was 160 mg%, and he made a face in response.

Christy looked at the number with concern. "What did we do wrong?"

"Bodine said all carbohydrates are not created equal," Gabe said. "I had about a cup of pasta and marinara sauce with my salad. I guess I'd better go running the next time I have pasta with tomato sauce. Meanwhile push-ups are probably my best option." He moved to the floor and began exercising. It amazed Christy that he could talk and work out at the same time.

"What are you doing?" he asked her.

"Making a list of the people I knew at the compound. I thought it might help."

"It might make a difference. They're going to have to look at all the bodies in the quarry lake." He sat up and lifted her chin to make eye contact.

"We should probably hit the trail in the morning. The longer we stay here, the more likely they are to come after us when we can't really hide. I've finished grading all the exams for my class and written the new lesson plans, so we're good to go for another week."

"Ask the agents about the witness program," Christy said. "Just to know."

"I did. Hawkeye said we aren't witnesses yet. Tracy's going to help push this through, and I know he'll do it. This will probably be our last week in the park." He dropped back into position and continued to exercise.

"I don't mind the park. I like spending the time with you and feeling like Adam and Eve. It's just thinking about the rest of it." She looked at him, pleading for understanding.

"I know, but just keep remembering we're getting the worst out of the way now."

"I'm remembering." She forced a smile. "I really am remembering. You were really awesome today. It was like watching a movie. It didn't even scare you, did it?"

"I'm one of those stupid people who gets off on adrenaline, but I promise to suppress the urge in the future. You know, I've been thinking about what Jonah said about Florida. He obviously doesn't think it will be permanent either, or he would have said Oklahoma and the Cherokee Nation. Living in Florida really wouldn't be bad. They've got springs there that are two-hundred-feet deep and crystal clear to the bottom. Some of them have unusual bacteria where the salt water from the ocean meets the fresh ground water. I'd like to see what sort of chemicals those little guys can break down. If they have the right biochemistry, they might teach us how to cure acid rain.

"I could teach you how to dive and then I'd have a permanent diving partner." He moved to sit beside her and ran his hand over her hair. "I'm really enjoying having you as my partner in everything else."

"I'd like to learn how to dive, but not like you did today. Jumping off the helicopter strut seemed a little extreme." She put her arms around him. "It scares me because I'm so afraid something will happen to you."

"I had to do a lot worse than that for a long time," he said.

"And you almost died. Reba told me how close you came to dying, Gabriel." She sat up and leaned over him. "I've lost all the people I've ever loved. I've never loved anyone as much as I love you."

"I'm being careful, Christy. To a trained diver, today wasn't a risk. You don't even want to know some of the places I've been as a Seal. Keep in mind I served in Desert Storm, and the Seal teams did some of the reconnaissance that told them where to bomb. The Iraqis were mining the Persian Gulf, and I had lots of fun locating mines and the boats that were carrying them. It was one time when my skin color was protection because I could pass for an Iraqi until I opened my mouth. I learned enough of the local dialects to say, 'drop your weapon and raise your hands.' I can do fairly well in German, Russian, and Spanish but not middle Eastern tongues." He smiled at her expression.

"I was on an anti-terrorism team after Desert Storm. On our safest missions, we were spies. We had to go into unfriendly territory and hope we could get out. If we didn't get out, it wasn't likely anybody would be able to come and get us. Four of the guys from my team are in the CIA now. Tracy was my commanding officer. If I hadn't gotten hurt, I would have had my own team. The Seals don't believe in rank giving you common sense, so everybody has the same training and the same requirements. There are two line officers on a team. One is the leader and the other is learning to lead."

"How did you get hurt when you're so good with guns and fighting?"

"I was dropped into battlefield situations. If I'm hunting the enemy, they're going to die. When they're hunting me, I can get hurt. I was shot in my right arm in Central America and broke my ankle on a jump in Caribbean. I got second degree burns on my face and hands on a mission in Lebanon. I was stabbed on a mission in Iraq. Almost every Seal I knew had more than one Purple Heart. There's so much risk involved that we take a medic and medical supplies with us as a part of the team. When I really got hurt, I went into fire to save Tracer. He would have been killed if I hadn't gone back for him.

"Looking back, I'd do it again even knowing the outcome because he's like a brother. I would have done it for anyone I served with. I can live with no peripheral vision better than I could have lived with his death from my cowardice. That's the only time I've ever invited trouble, and I wouldn't go into a dangerous situation again unless I had to do it to protect you. That's my job, and I'm going to do it." He kissed her with all of his deep feelings being transmitted in the kiss. In response, Christy stretched out on his body and held his wrists against the bed.

"I'm stronger than you think I am, and I'm going to protect you, too."

"And God is taking care of both of us," he added. That thought was the only reason he had been able to remain calm while the things he most cherished were threatened. Despite his faith, he didn't want to keep dwelling on the negative.

He kissed her while she still had his hands restrained and kept kissing her until her grip loosened and she let her hands slide down his arms to his chest. His dark eyes made her feel safe even before his arms were around her. Later, she fell asleep with her head on his chest and didn't dream.

When dawn broke, she was the first one dressed and packed. She completed her list while Gabe packed his gear and left it in the agent's hands as they stepped from the car. Oddly, she didn't feel any trepidation about the five days ahead of them. She was much more worried about what the following week would bring.

CHAPTER 20

As Seals, they had called premonitions of serious trouble, bad karma. Tracy and Gabe were both feeling it the next morning. In the kitchen, Tracy put his hand on Gabe's shoulder and said, "Hang tight. I'll bring the cavalry over the hill even if the feds won't."

The promise kept Gabe focused as they walked over the place where Darla had died in order to reach Hawkeye's car. The bad karma didn't ease despite the promise of reinforcements, but he had no doubts that Tracy Tolliver would keep his word. He didn't feel nearly as secure about the motives of the federal agents. He felt as if Hawkeye might be dangling them like bait to catch the biggest fish of his career.

Christy felt that Gabe seemed uneasy after they were dropped off in the national park. Even while they were in the car, he kept looking behind them as if he expected pursuit. They were taken to a road near Bryson City and left at a trail near the main highway. They spent the early part of the morning climbing down into a deep valley. Then Gabe kept them moving over the rocks and through the water to leave little or no trail as they walked deeper into the wilderness. He seemed to discourage conversation and stopped at intervals to listen to the woods around them. Christy kept her orientation by keeping the sun's position. She expected and needed to rest at noon, but Gabe just tossed her a bag of trail mix and kept moving.

At some point, the sun seemed to disappear though she was certain it was only early afternoon. There were very few clouds in the sky to block the sunlight, but the shadows seemed incredibly foreboding.

Christy was at her limit of endurance when Gabe propelled her up a rock face and through a maze of boulders. She was panting as they crawled into a narrow recess which widened into a cave. Gabe piled rocks in front of the opening and broke open a portable light source.

"We're being followed. They must have put a bug on Hawkeye's car because they've been following us since early this morning. Whoever it is knows how to track."

He opened his backpack and removed a bag she hadn't seen before then. As he reassembled it, Christy recognized a very specialized rifle.

"Is that what they call a sniper's rifle?"

"This is a sniper's rifle, and this is an laser scope. It lets me see day and night because it reads thermal images. If we're lucky, we might just capture some hired guns." He glanced at Christy. "Get some water and eat. We're going to be here awhile."

Awhile turned into the remainder of the day, but Christy vividly remembered the last time they had been attacked. She never questioned Gabe as he kept watch while lying on his abdomen on the rock floor. She watched for him when he had to pull off his fatigue jacket to stand the heat. It was very humid in the cave, and they went through their water supply rapidly. Late in the day, Gabe sent Christy back to see if there was a water source near them. She found a pool filling from a dripping spring and returned with a full canteen as he had directed.

"Keep watch for me," he whispered and put the rifle into her hands.

"I couldn't see any plants in the pool," Christy said nervously. "What about the springs you said didn't have visible life in them?"

"Out west some of the ground water is contaminated with arsenic," Gabe said. "If you see ground water with no life in it, you know you don't want to drink it. There isn't any plant life you can see in here because it's too dark." He took a box out of his backpack and filtered the water. Then he added a germicide to it. "This isn't going to be wonderful for our taste buds, but it will keep us from getting dehydrated." He took a long drink and then resumed his post. He gave the canteen to his wife.

"How did you learn all this?" Christy asked in fascination. "You're like an encyclopedia of Smoky Mountain survival techniques. Did they teach you all of this in the Navy?"

"I learned most of this before I enlisted. My grandfather, Gabriel, was a tribal elder. He used to take me up into 'the hills' as he called it. He never even finished high school because of being drafted into World War II, but he had learned what it took to survive here from his father and his grandfather. He was a part of these mountains, and he taught me that the Cherokee are a part of the earth. We don't think we own it or that it's ours to destroy. We're a part of it, so we should learn how to live with the land and care for it as if it were our mother. That was a part of the old ways, but it also fits everything I've read in the Bible.

"I think I believe the old ways were a gift from God, and the Native American peoples had the good sense to pass that wisdom down from father to son. My grandfather had knowledge in a way the scientists never will. He made me feel important because I was the vessel to carry his knowledge. I remember feeling like a sponge when I was with him. He died when I was fourteen, and even now I think of things I wish I had asked him. More than skin color, becoming one with the land is what made me Cherokee. Sometimes I take my questions to the tribal elders and write down everything I learn from them because every time one of them dies, the Cherokee people lose another volume of knowledge we'll never have again. Some archeologists believe the tribe has been here for ten thousand years. That's a huge heritage to lose. Do you remember what I told you about the original seven clans?"

"I remember you saying there were seven. Do you know which one you came from?" He glanced over at her and smiled.

"That's what I was going to tell you. They were called wolf, wild potato, deer, bird, long hair, blue, and paint. Most people don't know now because no records were kept about clanship, but both of my grandfathers knew. On my mother's side, we were descended from the paint clan. The Cherokee name was ANIWODI, and it was the clan most of the medicine men came from. They worked with plants to make their medicine.

"The old legend is that all diseases come from animals as revenge on man for killing them. The legend says the plants were friends to man because we cultivated them so for every disease that the animals give man there will be a cure from the plants. I've always thought my interest in plants might have been inherited from all the generations of the paint clan."

"That's really neat." Christy was fascinated. "What was your father's clan?"

"My grandfather Gabriel said his family was in the wolf clan. That was the clan most of the war chiefs came from. Obviously I inherited a certain amount of that side, too, and I did spend a couple of years being Chief Killian."

The conversation kept Christy from being afraid until the darkness continued to grow. Finally their sanctuary was swathed in shadows when Gabriel's watch said it wasn't yet night.

"Why is it so dark, Gabriel? Is there a storm coming?"

"We're in the Nantahala gorge," he said. "These caves were where the Cherokee hid from the soldiers to avoid the Trail of Tears. Nantahala is a Cherokee word. It means the land of the noonday sun. This gorge is so deep that the sun only shines into it when it's directly overhead."

Christy lay back and studied Gabriel's face. He showed no sign of being unnerved. She chose to take his assessment of the situation as her own. The advantage to their situation was being able to talk. She still found his every word to be fascinating.

"Did you go into the Navy because your father was in the Navy?"

"You're doing that ESP thing again," he said. "I took it really hard when my grandfather died. He was my connection to my father. At the time, I truly hated my mother. I couldn't reconcile how she could hug me and tell me she loved me and let Pritchard beat me half to death over and over again. I guess that's why mixed messages make me insane.

"I wasn't a Christian then so I couldn't relate to Jonah like I can now. I was dealing with a lot of negative feelings." He looked at Christy. "Remember what I told you about women being very important in Cherokee culture. By tradition, it should have been my mother's family that took me and raised me when she couldn't. When my mother was arrested, I was held at the base police station for three days while they tried to decide where I was going. I didn't know any of my father's family because I had lived at Virginia Beach all my life. We hadn't been back to Cherokee after my mother remarried. None of my mother's family would take me. Now I know they all had reasons. Her parents were both sick. Her father was dying from heart disease. Her mother had diabetes and was at her limit taking care of her husband. Her brother was an alcoholic and couldn't take care of his own family. Jonah and Reba came to get me. I remember sitting in the corner of a holding cell and seeing them for the first time. I knew they were there for me because they had the same skin color.

"They were strangers, and I didn't show any great gratitude to them for their trouble. I had had all the crying beaten out of me but not the anger. They hadn't been married very long, and I think Reba was about your age. She walked past all my hostility and picked me up. I could feel that they both cared about me from the first time they held me.

"For ten years they were my parents. I was an only child for three years, and then they had Naomi. Job came along when I was eleven. I almost could forget I didn't really belong in their home. They were my family, and they loved me as if I were really their son. When I was sixteen, my mother came home and expected me to move in with her. She wanted me to walk in the front door and pretend we'd always been together. I felt like it was my duty. I tried to talk to her. Then I tried to take care of her. I lasted in her house for three weeks, and then I lived in the woods. Love was Jonah and Reba hanging on to me when I was in court for truancy and in trouble for my mouth every other day.

"One day the Navy recruiter came to talk to the senior class, and I thought about my father and enlisted. Thank God, Jonah gave his permission. I guess I never felt like I belonged anywhere after my mother came home until I was a Seal. Some of the fault was mine for not being grateful for having a loving family. So God put me on my knees and kept me there until I had to look up."

Christy put her hand over his hand and held it. "We've been afraid of the same things. I was afraid of being alone and not being able to protect myself from the Divilbiss family because it was a situation I couldn't control. You were afraid of being alone and not being able to control diabetes. I'm not really afraid now. We can't control any of this, but really no one can control their life. They just follow the cloud or they stay lost. I'm not afraid to follow the cloud when I have you. I'll always be yours, and you'll always be mine." She could see him smile.

"I like that a lot better than until death do us part. When we have our big wedding, let's ditch that part of the vows. Forever is much more secure." Christy felt safe with her hand touching Gabriel despite their situation, and she fell asleep lying beside him. She awakened when the darkness in the cave seemed impenetrable. She couldn't see her husband anymore and had lost her grip on his hand.

"Gabriel, where are you?"

His hand came through the darkness and touched her lips. He moved until his lips were against her ear.

"Listen," he whispered. "You'll hear the crickets and frogs, and then they'll stop. The ones that tracked us are still out there so they must know we're somewhere in the rocks."

"What do we do?"

"Wait for them to make a mistake," Gabe said assuredly. "Be as quiet as you can."

Christy obeyed without question and ate a ration of food from their supplies without really tasting it. Afterwards she felt sick at her stomach and tried to sleep again without success. She crawled closer to Gabe and tried to see out into the night. He showed her the scope and pointed to a flickering light in the distance.

"They're camped over there. They don't care if we know where they are because they're pretty sure they know where we are. If I could get out of here without them seeing me, I'd take them out. I don't think I could defend shooting them with a sniper's rifle from here when they haven't fired on us. One of them is sitting guard duty."

"How can we get away?" Christy asked anxiously. "Can we call Hawkeye for help?"

"The radio won't receive inside the cave. When it's light outside they won't be able to see flares in here. We'll look for another way out. There are only two of them."

"Will there be another way out?"

"There almost always is," he whispered. "Listen, and you'll hear the bat wings. They aren't coming in past me, and they aren't trying to go out this way so they must have a back door." He squeezed her hand reassuringly as he saw her expression. "They aren't vampire bats, Christy. Vampire bats are only in South America. These little guys eat insects but not people."

"That's reassuring. I've already had enough vampire experience for one lifetime." She moved even closer until her body was against his. Even that contact made her feel more secure. It was cool in the cave, but his body warmth enveloped her. She could have slept again but could feel the tension in her husband's body and moved to rub his shoulders and back. Gradually she felt him relax.

"If you can't sleep, I may let you stand guard duty for a while," Gabe whispered. She realized he was tired and felt guilty for not offering to let him rest sooner.

"I can do it. Get some sleep."

"Don't try to take over my role. If you see anything, wake me up." His eyes told her the seriousness of the request, and she nodded.

"I will. I promise, Gabriel."

"Good girl." He rolled onto his back and put his arm over his eyes. She was sure he was asleep within minutes and decided that was probably a part of his training, too. The position of his arm made it possible for her to see his watch. The large iridescent dial was easy to read.

Christy let Gabe sleep from midnight until five o'clock. The flickering campfire had died out hours earlier, but the frogs and crickets told Christy that their stalkers weren't moving. When the forest was suddenly silent, she awakened Gabe hurriedly.

"They're moving."

He was back in position in an instant and took the rifle from her hands. Gabe could see the two men moving in the distance, but their camouflage made further details impossible. His eyes flickered toward Christy and told her to gather their gear. She was rolling up her sleeping bag when he suddenly scrambled away from the opening, carrying her with him and covering her body with his own. Their escape route exploded into a hail of rocks, mud, and debris.

Christy felt the impacts of many objects striking them through Gabe's body, and then there was darkness and complete silence. Gabe jerked once in response to an impact and then didn't move even when the debris had stopped falling on them. The weight of his body against her made it hard for Christy to breathe. She pushed him back with terror-driven strength and felt him roll limply to the floor of the cave.

It was hard to remember not to scream in fear and to move quietly. She was praying when she reached to feel his pulse and listened to see if he was breathing. She knew he was alive, but she couldn't see well enough to tell how badly he was hurt. She also knew she wasn't hurt because he had used his body to shield hers.

The sound of people climbing up the rock face took away her moment to gather her nerve. She snatched the handgun from Gabe's belt and climbed farther back into the cave. She took cover behind a huge boulder. She remembered to take off the safety and aimed the gun at the avalanche of loose rock. She could see the two sets of hands digging through the rocks. The hands were camouflaged green and brown.

"Let me be Deborah," Christy prayed. "Please don't let Gabriel die." She looked at her husband and suddenly was filled with rage because Divilbiss had hurt Gabriel. She had never fought back to protect herself, but she held the gun ready to kill anyone who came through the rocks.

Light poured into the cave as the men created an opening in the debris. Christy had one perfectly targeted, but she knew she needed to wait.

"We got them," the first man reported on seeing Gabe's body. "I'll check the ID, but the man looks like an Indian. He has a sniper's rifle next to him. It has to be Killian."

The second man appeared beside the first one, and Christy fired in their direction and kept firing. Her eyes were open the whole time, and she knew she had hit them. She kept firing to make sure they were dead, and the semiautomatic hand gun gave no pause between shots. Both men fell back and rolled down the rock face while Christy scrambled past Gabe to make sure they couldn't attack again. She looked down at the spreading blood across both men's bodies and tried not to gag. She had hit both of them in the chest more than once. She climbed back to Gabriel's side and began checking him for injuries as well as she could without turning him over again. She was afraid his neck or back might be hurt. When she found blood on the back of his head, she stopped looking for other injuries. She took the radio and called for help. Only static answered her. It occurred to her that the transmission might be blocked by the rock walls, and she ran to the mouth of the cave and used the radio again.

"Hawkeye, this is Windrunner. Come in, Hawkeye."

There was no answer, and Christy thought the radio must have been knocked off the correct frequency. She turned it off and returned to Gabe desperately. His face was still slack, and he was breathing convulsively. She stripped off the fatigue shirt over her tank top and soaked it with water from the canteen. She bathed Gabriel's face with the shirt and then shook him gently.

"Gabriel. Please wake up. Gabriel, you need to tell me what to do. Please wake up."

He stirred so slightly that for several moments Christy wasn't sure if she had imagined it. When his face contorted with pain, she was both relieved and frightened.

"Christy." He didn't open his eyes. "Don't let them get through the rock slide."

"It's okay," she said. "They're dead. I shot them with the handgun. Are you okay?"

"I'm not sure." Even opening his eyes seemed to be an effort, but he finally focused on her face. He lay very still as he sorted through the sensations in his body. Then he moved his hand slowly and felt his right side and his back. When he withdrew his hand, it was covered in blood. It was more blood than Christy had found on the back of his head. She could see a stream of it running out from under his body in response to his movement. She swallowed hard and started trembling as the reality of her husband's situation hit her.

"Shrapnel from the blast," he managed. "I saw them launch a grenade. You're going to have to get on the radio and get Hawkeye to help us."

"I tried," Christy said. "It wouldn't pick up. They wouldn't answer even when I used it outside."

"We're probably too low in the gorge. These rock faces can block the signal." He was silent as he struggled to breathe. "I don't know if I can walk out. I don't think I can." His eyes were on her face. "I love you, Christy."

She felt a cold wave of fear spread over her from her head to her feet because she knew he was telling her what she needed to hear in case he died.

"Help us, God," she prayed aloud. "Please help us get out of here." She kept praying silently for several minutes until she could feel her courage growing, powered by a force other than her will. She caressed Gabriel's forehead gently, not seeing how hard he was struggling to conceal his pain.

"I can climb to the top of the ridge and use the radio, Gabriel. What should it be set on?"

"21.5mHz," he said. "Let me look at it." She fumbled with the radio and put it in his hands. His hands were very unsteady, but Gabe managed to examine the radio. When he completed his inspection, he gave it back to her.

"It's set on the right frequency. It may be damaged, Christy. If it doesn't work on the ridge, you'll have to leave me and walk out to bring help. There's a ranger station about fifteen miles east of here. You can find it by using the compass until you can see the fire tower."

Christy looked at her husband and knew what he was suggesting would leave him defenseless and might leave him to die alone. She bent and looked at Gabe's watch. It was six o'clock in the morning.

"I can't leave you, Gabriel. I won't leave you. There has to be another way," she protested. "Do you have another one of those silver tarps? Should I cover the two bodies? It might reflect the light and let someone see us."

"It's in my backpack." He shifted position slightly and caught his breath to keep from crying out. As he became more fully conscious, the pain in his right chest was becoming almost unbearable. He clenched his fists in an attempt to hide it from Christy, but his face gave him away. Christy felt furiously angry because she was helpless to do anything for him. She wiped the blood off his hand and held both hands.

"Tell me what to do for you, Gabriel."

"I'm all right. We just need to get out of here." He looked at her, praying for control. "It's a hard climb to the top of the gorge. If you get hurt, there won't be a chance for either of us. It might be better if you just walk east and find the ranger station."

"I can climb out, Gabriel. I'm going to cover the bodies and start now."

"Go," he said tersely. "I'm okay." Before she could leave him, Gabe started shivering. Christy remembered the night she had been so sick from her infected leg. Instinct told her Gabe was going into shock.

"Should I try to stop the bleeding?" she asked with a tremor in her voice.

"There's something in my chest," he said. "If you pull it out, I might bleed even faster. It's probably better if I don't move because I could make it worse. When my pressure drops, the bleeding will slow down."

She pulled her sleeping bag over him and lay down beside him trying to warm him with her body. When she saw his lips were moving silently, she knew he was praying to hide his suffering from her. She wept silently as she held him.

"Stay with me, Gabriel," she whispered. "I love you."

"I'll be all right," he said for her sake. Though he was dazed from the blow to his head, Gabe knew he might not survive no matter what Christy was able to do. He spoke to try to alleviate her guilt in case he died. "If you can get help for me, I'll be all right for at least a few hours. If this were going to kill me right away, I'd already be dead. I may pass out if my pressure gets too low, but you'll still have time to get help. Remember life and death is in God's hands, Christy. If something happens to me, it was meant to happen."

"I can get help," she said fiercely. "I'm going to climb up the face and try the radio. If it won't work then, I'll hike until I find the ranger's station."

"You can do it. Don't be afraid." His pain began to ease, and Gabe relaxed his hands. As he stopped shaking, his body felt even colder to Christy. Despite his reassurances, she knew he was running out of time.

"I'm going now, Gabriel. Don't try to move." Christy took the hand gun and climbed down over the two dead men, swallowing hard when her stomach threatened to revolt. The easiest slope was almost straight up and studded with obstacles, but she didn't hesitate to start up it. It was a 250-foot climb.

"I can be Deborah," she repeated over and over. "I can be Deborah. God help me." Her booted feet slipped as she struggled for footing, and then she slid and just managed to catch a rock. She had to hold tightly and rest before her arms would allow her to move up again. She dared not look down because her fear of heights would have paralyzed her.

"God help me." She heaved her body upward again and thought of Gabe's clenched fists as he fought pain alone and with no hope of rescue. "God help me. Take care of Gabriel." She found another series of handholds and dragged herself up another twenty feet. The slope eased almost imperceptibly and allowed her to crawl up the last seventy-five feet. She had to pant to catch her breath when she reached the top. "Please, God. Let the radio work."

She flipped up the antenna and said, "Come in, Hawkeye. This is an emergency. Please come in, Hawkeye. This is Windrunner. We have an emergency."

"Go ahead, Windrunner," the agent's voice said. "What's the emergency?"

"We were attacked. Gabriel is hurt. It's very bad. We need a helicopter to get him to the hospital. Please hurry. He's in shock. Do you know where to find us? We're below these coordinates."

"I have you, Windrunner. We're coming. Hawkeye out."

She hurried down the mountainside sometimes sliding on her bottom and sometimes sliding on her stomach while clinging to the rocks. Gabe was lying very still when she reached him. Christy was frantic until she could touch him and feel he was still breathing. She bent close to his face.

"I got Hawkeye, Gabriel. He heard me. He said he's coming."

"That's good. You did good," he whispered. She could barely hear him, and she put her hand under the bedroll to hold him tightly. He was breathing very fast.

"I love you, Gabriel. Please stay with me. I really need you."

His hand was cold and damp, but it tightened over hers.

"I'm not going anywhere, baby. I can hang on until they get here." He paused to breathe and then continued, "The pain isn't so bad now. It's just hard to breathe." He paused to catch his breath again. "When we get back home, I need you to get on my laptop and send an e-mail to Tracy. His e-mail address is in my computer address book. Can you remember to do it?"

"I can remember," Christy vowed. "What should I tell him?"

"Just tell him what happened. He'll make sure you're safe until I can." Gabe was speaking with great effort, and Christy had to bend close to hear his last words, "Promise me."

"I promise, Gabriel." She moved behind him and put his head in her lap in an effort to make him more comfortable. She kept the gun beside her leg ready to fight to the death to defend him. She pressed her hands against his face, and he looked into her eyes as long as he could. His last conscious thought was a prayer for Christy.

She couldn't let herself realize he was unconscious, and she told him her dreams of their future because they seemed so tenuous.

"When you're better, I want to have your baby, Gabriel. I've always wanted to have three or four children and a big yard full of flowers, but I didn't think it would happen until I met you. I can close my eyes and see our babies. They're going to have your eyes. I love your eyes, Gabriel. In the summer, we can lay out in the back yard and look at the stars." She wiped her eyes with one hand to keep her tears from falling on his face.

"I love you, Gabriel." When she put her hand his face again, she felt no response to her touch. She knew he was unconscious and maybe dying. Then she prayed out loud saying all the memorized prayers she had ever heard along with simple pleas for her husband's life. It became harder to keep praying when she realized Gabe's color was growing dusky. His pulse was too rapid for her to count.

"Please, God," she begged. "Please let them come in time. I'll never ask for anything again if you'll let Gabriel live." She hadn't known she could love someone so much as she sat fearing he would die.

CHAPTER 21

It was a long time before she heard the helicopter, and at first she wondered if she had imagined it. Gabriel's watch told her it was almost nine o'clock, enough time for Hawkeye to have arranged such specialized transport and to have located them. When she was certain it was a helicopter, she hurried out of the cave to make certain they knew where to come. The agent had obviously seen the bodies, and he stood on the strut directing the helicopter until it could descend straddling the stream. Christy went back to Gabe and hurriedly broke down his rifle so she could hide it in his backpack. She had just completed the task when two men dressed as paramedics climbed into the cave and pushed her aside. Gabe made no response to their examination. Christy swayed when she saw the pool of blood under her husband. A piece of wood was extending out of his chest.

"Get the basket," one of the paramedics shouted. "He's in deep shock. We need to get him out of here *now.*"

She was praying again while they cut the branch off flush against Gabe's chest and then covered the wound.

Gabriel was lifted into a basket and carefully carried down the rock face. Christy gathered all their gear and then struggled to shoulder the weight. She had to drag it down the cliff to keep her balance. By the time she climbed into the helicopter, her husband was covered with life-support equipment. On the monitor, his heart rate was 170, and his blood pressure was only 70/40 despite the rapid infusion of intravenous fluids into both of his arms. An oxygen mask covered most of his face, keeping Christy from the reassurance of seeing him. The paramedics allowed her to sit close to Gabe with her hand on his shoulder as they took off. His words did nothing to reassure her.

"This is your husband?" Christy nodded. "I need his full name."

"It's Gabriel W. Killian."

"How old is he?" the paramedic asked matter-of-factly.

"He's thirty-one. His date of birth is September 1, 1967." Christy closed her other hand over the silver cross around her neck and held it as a prayer.

"What race?" the paramedic asked as he continued down his checklist.

"He's a Cherokee." She glanced over the clipboard and saw the paramedic check the box marked 'other.' She started crying silently. She had never felt more alone.

"Any medical problems?"

"He has diabetes and high blood pressure," Christy said. She shuddered when she saw the paramedic's expression.

"Any allergies?"

Christy didn't know, but she took the dog tags from her shirt and looked at them. "I'm not sure, but it would be on his dog tags if he were, wouldn't it?"

The paramedic shook his head. "I don't know, ma'am. Is he active duty?"

"No. He's been out for four years." They were clearing the mountaintops, and the paramedic questioning her got on his radio.

"Mercy Trauma, this is mobile rescue one. We're transporting a Native American man aged thirty-one. He was injured in an explosion and has a projectile in his right posterior chest. He has no breath sounds over his right chest. His pressure is 75/45 and his heart rate is 160. I have two lines of LR going wide open. He's on a 100% face mask with an O2 saturation of 85%. He's had extensive bleeding from the chest wound. I'd estimate at least four units. There's also a scalp laceration over his occipital scalp. He's unresponsive to any stimuli."

"Mobile rescue one, what's your ETA?" the radio asked.

The paramedic scanned the horizon. "ETA is thirty minutes, Mercy Trauma."

Christy reached past the paramedics to touch Gabe's face above the oxygen mask. "Will he be okay?"

The paramedic looked at her sympathetically. "He's hurt pretty bad, ma'am, but I've seen people hurt a lot worse that did just fine."

Hawkeye examined the two bodies during the first fifteen minutes of their flight. During the last twenty minutes, he moved to question Christy.

"I need to know what happened, Mrs. Killian."

Christy looked at the agent and then quickly back to Gabe. "He knew someone was following us. We took shelter in the cave, and we could see them all through the night. Gabe had said we would try to explore the cave and find another way out at dawn, but they threw a grenade at us. Gabe saw them throw it and covered me with his body. I felt everything hitting us. It seemed to last forever, and when it was over Gabe was unconscious. I got his gun and hid behind some rocks. When they dug into the cave to get us, I shot at them. I just kept on shooting. I didn't know what else to do. They knew who we were. They called Gabriel by name."

"You did just fine," Hawkeye replied soothingly. "I'm pretty sure the blond-haired man is on the fifty most wanted list. I didn't know you knew how to shoot."

"Gabriel taught me," she said slowly. "And I prayed. I prayed really hard. Like I'm praying now."

Hawkeye put a comforting hand on her shoulder and gave her a tissue to wipe the tears she couldn't feel. As Hawkeye sat back, he was feeling the need to avenge a man he was starting to consider a comrade in arms.

They were airlifted to the trauma center at Mercy Hospital, and Hawkeye stayed with Christy when the trauma team took Gabe and ran with him. The worst moment of the waiting was when the nurse brought her Gabriel's watch, wedding ring, and his silver cross.

Christy's hands were shaking when she signed the papers giving them consent to take her husband to surgery. She spent the rest of that day on her knees in the waiting room. At six o'clock that night, the surgeon came to talk to her and helped her sit down.

"I'm Dr. Peterson, Mrs. Killian. Your husband is in intensive care. He had a long piece of wood entering his right back. It had collapsed his right lung. We opened his chest and cleaned out the foreign bodies. We repaired his lung, and he has a chest tube in place to reinflate it. He was on the ventilator until just a few minutes ago when I was able to extubate him. Right now he's breathing well on his own. He had a cut on the back of his head, and I'm sure he has a concussion, but the CT scan looks good aside from his old injury. Other than that, he took some blunt trauma to his back and legs but none of those injuries are serious. He bled out about half his blood volume from a torn bronchial artery, but I didn't transfuse him yet. We've given him enough plasma expander to bring his blood pressure to normal. He has a rare blood type, and we don't have any matching units here or at the blood bank. There was a multiple trauma two days ago that used every unit of his type in the city. They're calling for donors, but it takes time. I can give him O- if I have to..."

"He's AB-. So am I," Christy interrupted. "You can take my blood for him. He donated blood for me once, so we're compatible. I've given blood before, and I know you can take more in a few days if you have to."

"The one unit will be plenty for now," the doctor assured her. "He's young and strong. He can handle having a hematocrit of 20% or more. Right now his count is 17%, and that kind of anemia puts anyone in low grade heart failure. It's a little more of a stress when the patient is already breathing off one lung instead of two." He gestured to a nurse. "Call the blood bank and ask them to come over here for an emergency donor directed transfusion. His wife is AB- too."

"Not many guys are smart enough to carry their own blood supply," the nurse said as she smiled.

"Probably more people do it than anyone imagines," Christy replied grimly.

"There's one other thing," Dr. Peterson said. "Your husband's blood sugar was a little over two hundred on arrival. Is he diabetic?"

"He was just diagnosed," Christy said. "He gets checked for it every year at the VA. He tests it at least once a day, and all the ones after meals are under 140 unless he eats something high in carbohydrates. Our educator said that was good. He takes an ACE inhibitor for his blood pressure and a statin drug for cholesterol."

"Right now he's going to need insulin. We have to keep him in the normal range, or he'll be at a much greater risk for infection and poor healing. The human immune system doesn't work as it should when the blood sugar is out of normal range."

"Does that mean he will need insulin forever? Isn't that bad?"

"No," the doctor said soothingly. "Insulin isn't addictive so lots of diabetics take it for a while and then get off it. Taking insulin doesn't mean the diabetes is more serious. Diabetes is diabetes. If your sugar is in control, it's good. When your sugar isn't controlled, you put the 'die' into the diabetes. I'll ask one of the endocrinologists to see him. He really should be on an insulin sensitizer because Native Americans are very resistant to insulin, just like African Americans. Those drugs have been shown to help protect how much insulin a diabetic can make on their own, and they will probably lower the risk of heart disease."

"It's very new to me," she said, "and I'm very afraid for him. Do whatever you have to do to make him well."

Christy scarcely felt the needle they put in her arm, and she wouldn't have cared if it had hurt. She focused on the memory of Gabriel's face until the phlebotomist had completed her task.

"Your blood count is a little low, honey," the tech told her. "You might want to take some iron. You were running 34% before this donation. I couldn't have taken your blood if it weren't an emergency."

Christy nodded acceptance of the recommendation and thought of her blood count before Gabe had given her blood. She drank the three containers of juice Hawkeye brought her and then went to the pay phone to call Jonah and Reba. She asked them to bring Gabriel's laptop. They arrived just after she was allowed to see Gabriel for the first time.

Gabe was still on the oxygen mask, but her blood was being run into his vein, and his face looked less dusky. His eyes were closed.

"I love you, Gabriel," she whispered. "I really love you so much."

"I love you, too," she heard him say. "I'm okay, Christy."

She held his left hand between both of hers and kissed it. His fingertips caressed her cheek. "The doctor says you're going to be all right."

"I knew you'd take care of me," he said. "Did you get Tracer?"

"I will. I'll get him in just a little while." She caressed the straight dark hair from his forehead and felt him relax under her hand. The nurse let her stay beyond the actual visiting time, and she left the ICU accompanied by Hawkeye.

Jonah and Reba were in the waiting room and came to meet her immediately. "How is he?"

"He's out of surgery, and the doctor says he's doing well. He could talk to me."

"He'll be all right," Reba assured her. "God saved Gabe for a purpose, Christy, and I know he won't be taken now. You know he was named for an angel." She opened her Bible to the first chapter of Luke and showed Christy the nineteenth verse which read, "I am Gabriel who stands in the presence of God." Christy traced the verse with her fingertips and thought of seeing Gabriel in the woods with the light illuminating his face like a halo.

"He's been my angel." She burst into tears despite trying not to show how she felt. Jonah and Reba held her arms in support as they were taken to a private family waiting room Hawkeye had arranged. Twenty tissues later she used the telephone line and electric outlet to send the e-mail to Tracy Tolliver. When she signed off the internet, she noticed a letter to Job on the desktop and opened it. The letter helped her make it through the night.

Job, I had to write you because I don't know what may happen with me and Christy. Everything has been changing so fast, but the changes have been good for me. My only regret is knowing how you've suffered over losing Darla. I wish I could make you know that joy can still come in the morning like your dad always told us. I kept waiting and finally the joy came for me when I didn't expect it. I love you, Job. You've been my brother instead of my cousin. You knew I needed you so when I felt the most alone, you came and were there without asking questions or wanting answers. That's a great gift. It's the gift your father has, and he gave it to you. I think God expects us to use our gifts so He must have tremendous confidence in you.

I've told your father that we may have to go in the witness protection program. If we do, I'll make sure you know we're okay, and someday we'll be able to look back on these years and know it was when we both grew up.

Gabe

Christy had to swallow hard as she closed the computer. Jonah came to sit beside her in the quiet darkness and took her hand.

"I think of Gabriel as my son. His father and I were very close. The worst day of my life was when they said my brother was dead. It was harder than losing our father because he had lived a long life. Adam was only twenty. When Reba and I were asked to take Gabe, it was like an answer to my prayers to have my brother back. Of course, it wasn't like that. I was very young then, and Gabe was a very angry child. I have prayed more for Gabe than my other two children, and God answered my prayers. He has grown into the kind of man every man wishes his son to be. He is sometimes very impulsive, but he always prays before he makes decisions now.

"I know he loves you very much. I was worried at first because your relationship happened so suddenly. Now I really believe God put the two of you together, and I'm not worried about him any more. You shouldn't be either. He has a mission in this life, and I know he'll live to carry it out with your help."

Christy wiped her eyes and forced a smile. "I was so afraid this would happen. I held back from how I felt about him because I was afraid he would get hurt. I wish it had been me."

"The world is under God's direction, Christy. Sometimes it doesn't seem so, but I know it is. This is a message to point you both in another direction. If Gabe was meant to die, he would be dead. Keep your heart open, and God will tell you what to do next." She held Jonah's hand a long time, and finally she was able to sleep.

CHAPTER 22

Commander Tracy Tolliver appeared at the door to the intensive care unit in civilian clothes but accompanied by several other naval officers. He caught Christy's arm as she and Jonah came out of the unit.

"Is Gabe all right?" he demanded. Christy nodded because at first she didn't trust herself to speak without bawling.

"He's still having a hard time breathing, and he's in a lot of pain. The doctor says he's going to make it." Her voice broke, and Tracy put a protective arm around her shoulders.

"I won't let anything else happen to you," Tracy asserted. "This business has gone on long enough. I want to see what the federal people have got going, and then if they don't press on, I'm going to turn up the heat under them." He took Christy's arm. "Come on back to the waiting room. I brought in some food. You look like you could use it."

The Chinese food Tracy had brought didn't even smell appealing to Christy. She had a hard time making herself eat and then felt sick again. The nausea hit her in a sudden wave and made her run for the ladies' room. She was sitting on the floor still heaving when Reba handed her a wet paper towel and tied back her long hair.

"Christy, could you be pregnant? You remind me of how I was when I was expecting Job and Naomi." Christy tried to take slow deep breaths as she counted the time in her head. When she realized what Reba was suggesting could be true, she felt the blood rush to her face.

"Maybe. I hadn't thought about it. I didn't have time to think about it. My cycle should have been Friday." She pressed the towel to her mouth. "It would have happened right after we got married." Reba smiled and passed Christy another towel.

"Sometimes it happens faster than you think it will, but it's always God's will. I'm going to get you some soda to settle your stomach. Just sit there until I get back."

Christy nodded and leaned against the wall with her eyes closed. Her stomach was still churning, and when she thought of being pregnant amid so much turmoil, she felt even worse. They hadn't really talked about having children except on their wedding night when they had made the snap decision not to worry about birth control. As Christy remembered that night, she thought of Gabe saying, "I hope we are making a baby." The memory eased the tension inside her and allowed the nausea to lessen.

The bathroom door opened and closed to allow Reba to leave. Christy focused on breathing slowly and deeply, trying to ignore the angry voices of Tracy and Hawkeye. She moved her hand slowly down to touch her abdomen and smiled involuntarily as she thought of Gabriel. It was comforting to think she might have some part of him inside her body.

"Maybe it's a sign from God that we're done with all the worst times," she thought. "I'm not going to tell Gabriel until I'm sure." She heard the door open and said, "Reba? Don't tell Jonah yet. I don't want to tell Gabriel until I'm sure."

Something inside Christy told her the door had admitted someone other than Reba. She came to her feet and slammed the stall door as hands tried to grasp her. She started screaming at the top of her lungs and pressed herself into the corner of the stall. The door was kicked open and a gun was shoved into the stall.

"Shut up!" the woman demanded. "Now you're going to walk out of here like we've been best friends all our lives."

Christy nodded mutely and managed to walk slowly toward her captor as she tried to remember the martial arts moves Gabe had taught her.

"Put your arms around my waist," he had ordered her. Then he feigned stepping back on her foot followed by a hard elbow to her abdomen and a final blow to her face. Of course, he hadn't ever really hit her, but he had made her hit him when they practiced to show her how to land the blows. "Those three blows will buy you enough time to run." He had made her practice them over and over again.

Christy and her captor reached the bathroom door as Reba returned. When Reba pushed open the door, Christy breathed a prayer and stomped on the woman's foot. The second and third blows were automatic, and the gun clattered across the bathroom floor. Christy screamed and tried to get through the door as her captor recovered and wrestled her to the ground. They were struggling when Hawkeye threw the door open and tackled the woman, pinning her to the tile floor.

"Search the rest of the hospital," he ordered his men. "Get security to seal off this wing and call the local police. This lady needs to pay a visit to the local jail, don't you, sweetheart?" He jerked the woman to her feet while Reba remained on the floor beside a shaken Christy. Tracy helped both of them up and walked them back to the family room. He and the other naval officers stood guard around Gabe's family for the remainder of the day. They even followed Christy to the nurses' lounge and kept watch while she showered and changed her clothes.

Christy walked back to the ICU every visiting interval and always felt relieved on seeing Gabriel's face. At the last visit that day, he had been taken off the oxygen mask and was using only the nasal oxygen. His eyes were on Christy from the moment she reached the door to his room, and he reached out his left hand to her. She could tell he was really awake for the first time since his injury.

"I hope you brought my wedding ring. I feel undressed without it." The words were light hearted and made Christy smile as she took his cross and ring out of her pocket.

"It feels good to put it back on your hand," she said as she slipped the band on his finger. He took her hand.

"Keep my cross until I get out of here. It might get tangled up in all this technology. The nurses told me you donated the blood I got. I'll bet you didn't tell them you were profoundly anemic when you were in the hospital a little over two weeks ago."

"My blood count was 34%," she reassured him. "This time you needed it more than I did. I gave it without gas or anything to help me with the needle. Loving somebody is a great anesthetic." She held his hand against her body. "You scared me, Gabriel. I hadn't ever been that scared." His eyes caressed her.

"I know it was bad for you, baby, but you did it. You did everything right. You earned your Seal dog tags." His eyes were anxious. "They won't let me out of intensive care until tomorrow morning. Did Tracer come?"

"He's been here kicking Hawkeye's butt at every opportunity. He brought a whole bunch of Navy guys with him."

"Navy officers might be a better description." His dark eyes scanned her face with concern. "Stay with Tracy, Christy. He'll make sure nobody bothers you. You look pale. You really shouldn't have donated that blood. Are you okay?"

"I'm locked into the Deborah mode," she reassured him. "I'm going to take good care of you until it's your turn to take care of me again. I wish they'd let me stay with you."

"If they don't tomorrow, I'm going to pitch a fit. I probably can't pitch it very far, but I'm still going to try." He shifted position and grimaced. "I think I've passed you in being sore." She bent to kiss his forehead, but Gabriel was quicker and kissed her lips.

"You're better medicine than anything they're giving me."

"That goes both ways." She glanced at the nurse who was obviously awaiting her departure. "I know. Time to go. I love you, Gabriel. Try to be a patient patient."

"I'm trying. Believe me." He waited until the nurse stepped back out and said, "Are you sure you're okay? You look different somehow."

"I'm sure. I'm just worried about you." Letting go of his hand was the hardest part, and she released him very reluctantly. As she walked out of intensive care, she felt like running back but knew it would serve no purpose. Two police officers met her at the door and escorted her to the family room.

Reba and Jonah had taken a hotel room down the street and returned with ginger tea and biscuits to feed Christy. Surprisingly both seemed to settle her stomach. When Jonah was talking to one of the policemen, Reba slipped a boxed pregnancy test into Christy's hands and propelled her toward the door. She was followed to the bathroom by the officers and felt self conscious when she went inside to read the box. The test strip turned pink almost immediately. The box called pink positive.

Christy's face was almost the same color as the test strip when she returned to the waiting area. Reba's smile was very reassuring.

Tracy came to question her about Gabriel's condition with genuine concern and then showed his relief when Christy gave her report.

"Gabe was always kind of a loner. I've known him since he was twenty and I was twenty-two. We did Seal training together, and we got to be friends then. He asked to be assigned to my team when we came out of training, and we worked together for seven years."

"He gave one hundred ten percent to everything we did, and he was the best at a lot of things. The teams cross train so every man knows something about the other specialty jobs. Gabe was the best in martial arts and absolutely the best with weapons. Some men with those talents get to be arrogant, but Gabe never was. He just did his job no matter what it took. He got hurt three times that I remember, and every time he was hurt, it happened because he was helping another team member.

"Before he went to OCS, he was a Chief Petty Officer, and the Navy refers to those officers as Chief and their last name. Imagine being a Native American and being called Chief. Some of the other guys gave him trouble about being Cherokee because they were envious of how far he had made it up the career ladder. He took the constant hazing when most of us would have fought back. I was the team leader, and I liked him, but I didn't stand up for him when I should have.

"When he came back from officer's candidate school, he was over the guys who had hazed him. You never would have known it by how he acted. He was a team player and a team leader. After a while, he earned the respect of every member of every team.

"The day Gabe got hurt, we were doing reconnaissance in a very unfriendly country in South America. The carrier inserted the team at a commercial harbor, and we entered through a dock. After we did our business, we came back to the dock so we could swim out to the extraction point. The wrong people saw us and followed us. We met heavy resistance while we were running for the water. We knew if we made it to the water we could get to the extraction point. Gabe was on the point, and he stopped and covered the first four guys of the eight man team until they were in the water. I was covering the back, and when I started to move up, I was hit in the leg. Gabe got the other three into the water and called for a hot extraction. Then he came back for me. None of the others even tried.

"There were five guys pursuing us. Gabe shot four of them before he got to me. The fifth one shot him, but Gabe still engaged him in hand to hand combat while I crawled across the dock to get in the water. I didn't even know Gabe had been hit until later. He was actually hurt worse than I was even then, but he kept fighting until I was in the water. I yelled for him to extract, and he broke away. The other guy tackled him when he was running, and they fell off the dock together and dropped fifteen feet to the shore. I was waiting for him in the water, and I heard them hit the rocks. The other guy was killed by the fall.

"I thought Gabe was dead when I got to him. I dragged him out into the harbor because I didn't want to leave his body. He was just about dead by the time they got us out. The commander had to airlift him in a combat helicopter to get him to Florida fast enough to save him. These other guys were a part of that team, and we all know what would have happened to us if Gabe Killian hadn't sacrificed himself. After that, I understood why they used to call Indian men braves. I'll bet he never told you how he got hurt."

"That wasn't the story he told me. He said you were extracting under fire, and when he was shot he fell off the dock."

238   *Terri Wood Jerkins*

"That's my definition of heroic," Tracy said. "Risking your life for someone else and then feeling no need to brag about it. He would tell you that he just did his duty."

"Gabe saw them throw a grenade at us, and he covered me with his body," Christy said quietly. "If he hadn't, I might be in intensive care. Thank you for coming, Tracy. It will mean a lot to Gabe. He talks about you all the time."

"Not many people are lucky enough to have a friend like Gabe. I'll be here as long as he needs me to be."

As the next visiting hour approached, Reba whispered, "I think you should tell Gabe about the baby. He'll be so excited, it will make everything else easier. Gabe loves kids, and he's really good with them." Christy was bursting with the secret, and Reba's words made the decision for her.

Hawkeye detained her from going just as the visiting hours were announced. "We need to talk first, Mrs. Killian. We have some new information from the woman we arrested."

"Did she tell you who hired her?" Christy asked.

"She's willing to make a deal. She has a very long rap sheet. She knows if you press charges, she'll probably get a long sentence because she'll be classed as a habitual criminal. She knows she was hired by someone in the Divilbiss corporation. Since Carlton Divilbiss is the CEO, we can charge him. That and your testimony before a grand jury should give us enough evidence to go into the compound."

"I'll do whatever you think I should do," Christy said. "Just get these people before they kill anyone else."

"Promising to testify makes you a witness," Hawkeye said soothingly, "and we can get you and Dr. Killian out of here." That knowledge was a blessing and a curse, but Christy thought of how much at risk Gabriel was and nodded.

"We'd like to go to central Florida where the Seminole tribe is."

"Good choice," Hawkeye told her. "I was afraid you would ask to go to the Cherokee Nation in Oklahoma, and that will be the first place they will look for you. I'll see if we can't get a grand jury convened. We're going to keep plenty of guards on both of you because you're our main witness. All the rest of our case is circumstantial, but we can link it to Divilbiss with your help. Ballistics has matched the bullets that killed those six hikers to the guns on the men you killed. With that and this woman's testimony, we have conspiracy to murder and seven counts of first-degree murder. Even with expensive lawyers, Divilbiss is going to prison at the very least.

"Just get the other people out, Hawkeye," Christy said pleadingly. "Don't let them kill the others."

CHAPTER 23

Gabe experienced three days of feeling dazed and sedated. The concussion he had suffered kept his memory and time relationships muddled until the fourth morning when the doctor said he would be moved from intensive care. That morning the reality of being unable to protect Christy and himself began to hit. He was dwelling on that when Hawkeye appeared at his door.

"I suppose you've come for a chorus of 'I told you so,'" Gabe said. "If I had had a kevlar vest, this would have played out differently."

"Actually I came to congratulate you and to take your statement," Hawkeye said. "I lost a fifty dollar bet on you. I didn't think you'd last a week, and I didn't know they would use grenades." Gabe smiled slowly.

"Knowing you lost the bet will make this part easier."

Hawkeye sat down beside the bed. "I think we have enough evidence to convene a grand jury. It would be safer for you and your wife if you entered the federal witness protection program."

"I know," Gabe said. "I figured that out while I was staring at them through my gun sight. I knew I could easily kill them. I wanted to pull the trigger, but I didn't because that wouldn't end this. It was a lot easier when I could take the law into my own hands."

"Your wife said they stalked you all morning and held you at bay in the cave where we found you."

"I thought they would give up, but it got dark and they were still watching the cave. I knew they'd see a flare if we tried to look for another way out. At sunrise they launched a grenade at us. I saw it. I had time to cover Christy. That's all I remember."

"Apparently you aren't a bad teacher. Your wife shot both of them three times in the chest. They never knew what hit them. If you stayed out in the park, we might get rid of every paid assassin in this country."

"You have a perverse sense of humor, but I'm sure I'm not the first to recognize it." Gabe closed his eyes. "I'm stuck with trusting you for now."

"I can keep you safe, Dr. Killian. You have my word on it. Just rest and get over this. We need you and your wife to get these vultures. When they discharge you, we'll get you out of the state. There are guards on your wife constantly now."

Christy was feeling relieved even before the nurses came to tell her Gabriel had been moved to the trauma floor. Before she could go visit him, Dr. Peterson came to meet with her and introduced Dr. Shepherd, an endocrinologist.

"He's coming along very well, Mrs. Killian," Dr. Peterson said. "His blood count came up over 20% after the unit you gave him, and he's almost off oxygen. From my standpoint, the worst is over." He looked at the diabetes specialist who stepped forward.

"Unfortunately, his blood sugar hasn't returned to normal. He's going to need medication to control it and possibly insulin for a another few days. Diabetes frequently appears when people are under stress, and it's obvious he's been under some stress. It's very common in Native Americans, as I'm sure you know. In the tribes we've studied, there are genetic defects that predispose them to getting diabetes.

"I'm starting your husband on a medicine called Avandia. It makes people with type 2 diabetes more sensitive to insulin, and it seems to preserve what insulin making cells they have left if we start it soon enough. When people are near ideal body weight and still develop diabetes, it means they don't have many insulin making cells left. This drug works better than anything else to preserve how much insulin he has left. All the studies done on this drug indicate it will probably cut his risk of heart disease. It seems to work against every negative risk factor diabetes carries.

"There are a few precautions you need to know about. This class of drug can make it easier for people to gain weight especially if they eat fat. Avandia works by making fat go into fat cells. Since fat circulating in the blood stream damages the blood vessels, we want it to drive fat into the fat cells. The downside is if a person takes the drug and eats a high fat diet, they can gain weight. I think you both know that fat is the worst thing he could eat, and I've warned him as well. He will also need to have his blood drawn to test his liver every two months for the first year he's on the drug. It hasn't shown any tendency to hurt the liver, but another drug in the family did.

"The last warning is that people can retain fluid when they take Avandia. You may even hear people say that it can cause heart failure. If a person on the drug develops heart failure, it's because they already have a weak heart muscle and retained fluid. We think it may keep hearts healthy if we use it soon enough. All people with diabetes retain salt easily because the hormones in the body that cause salt retention get turned on by diabetes.

This drug can sometimes make that worse. We give the drug at supper to decrease the fluid retention. My experience has been that people do not swell unless they eat too much salt. I would want to know if he did develop any swelling so I could decrease the dose."

Christy nodded as if she weren't overwhelmed by her fears for Gabriel. She was still feeling as if she were being swept downstream by white water when Marilyn Cooper came to meet with her.

"I'm one of the diabetes educators, Mrs. Killian. I've been meeting with your husband. He thought you might have questions for me."

"I have so many that I don't know where to begin asking," Christy said. "The diabetes doctor said Gabe is going to need insulin. I guess I don't understand why. The educator in Asheville says he had type 2 diabetes. He said that's the non insulin dependent kind. Why does he need insulin?"

"The stress of his injuries has caused his body to make steroid hormones that make him even more resistant to insulin. Now he can't generate enough insulin to keep his blood sugar normal. It is critically important to keep him in the normal range now to reduce his risk of infection and promote healing. He should be able to come off insulin when the stress resolves. Most type 2 diabetics need supplemental insulin when they are seriously ill."

"Does he have any other damage from the diabetes?" Christy asked. "Will this make him worse?"

"He has no signs of damage at all," Marilyn said. "Your husband has completely normal eyes. We had retinal photographs taken to be certain. He has no signs of cataracts and no protein in his urine. Our CT scanner here can look for coronary lesions, and he's already had two scans with no evidence of any heart disease. He's lucky to know about it before he had developed any damage.

"You're lucky that he's so motivated to do every-thing the right way. He says you know about blood pressure and lipids. He needs a blood test on his lipids and blood sugar every three months. The test to check his blood sugar is called a glycohemoglobin or HgbA1C. That measures how much sugar or glucose is attached to the hemoglobin in his blood. If he has 7.0% or less, the American Diabetes Association considers him to be in excellent control. That number can't be too low because it's just the tip of the iceberg when it comes to changes in the proteins in his body. People without diabetes run 4% to 6%.

"He needs an eye examination every year, and he needs a urine test to check his kidneys every year. He already knows how to draw and give insulin because of his mother. I'm going to teach you how to draw and give insulin and how to give the antidote to insulin. That's called glucagon. If someone has a low sugar from insulin, a shot of glucagon will bring their sugar back to normal. People with type 2 diabetes don't usually have low blood sugars, but they can when they are on insulin sensitizers with insulin. A low sugar is a reading under 60 with symptoms. People don't pass out from a low sugar unless they are under 40, and that's very uncommon in type 2 diabetics who don't take insulin."

Christy spent an hour with the educator and was given several books to read. As they finished, one of the volunteers came to escort her to Gabe's new room. He was sitting upright in bed and smiled at her. She knew him well enough to see the undercurrent of tension in his eyes.

"I'm doing great. How are you?"

"A lot better now." She exhaled her relief and entered the room to sit on the edge of the bed. It was comforting just to hold both his hands. "Hawkeye is convening a grand jury. He thinks it will be soon, and since I'm his main witness that's going to put us in the federal witness

protection program. I told him central Florida." Gabriel's
face showed nothing but relief.

"I'm glad. I probably won't be able to finish my
classes anyway, and these people are ruthless. It would
be different if we could just go after them, but the law
protects them as much as it protects us. I wish we could
leave now. Is Tracer keeping you safe?"

"I'm here, aren't I? I have a whole bunch of guards
around me all the time." She sat back and looked at him
almost timidly. Suddenly it didn't seem easy to tell her
husband he was going to be a father when she had only
known him a few weeks.

"You've got that weird look again," Gabe said.
"What's wrong, Christy?"

"Nothing's wrong," she stammered. "Gabriel, I'm
pregnant. Reba brought me a test, and I'm sure. I know
the timing isn't good." She held her breath until she saw
the elation on his face.

For Gabe, her words were the answer to his prayer.
He knew that they needed to leave, and knowing his
family was at stake made the decision to go much easier.
He was certain it hadn't happened by chance.

"Really, Christy? You're sure?" He pulled her into
his arms and held her as if they weren't in his hospital
room. "I just can't believe it happened so quick. I know
you probably would have preferred it happen later, but
it's great. It's like a sign from God that He's blessing us
being together. Don't get out of the guards' sight for a
second, Christy. Not even a second. Promise me." She
felt elated because of his response and couldn't stop
smiling.

"They're following me to the bathroom, Gabriel. Can
I at least close the stall door?"

He laughed and grimaced with the pain that followed. "You can close the stall door, but they had better
be outside. I can't tell you how much better you've made
me feel. I really needed a way to get refocused. Since I

started waking up, I've felt like a prisoner. Hawkeye promised he can keep us safe when we leave here. It's time for me to get moving. They pulled the chest tube this morning."

"Gabriel, please don't push yourself," she begged. "I need you to be able to take care of me for the long haul. I don't know how long I can stay in the Deborah mode."

Gabe sat forward and put his legs off the bed. He felt very dizzy for several moments, and the dizziness controlled him when the pain didn't. Christy felt dizzy for him when she saw his back. The neat bandage was not what horrified her. Even his dark skin couldn't conceal the many bruises that extended from his shoulders to his hips. She remembered feeling the blows through his body. She knew he had taken those blows to save her. She sat down behind him and caressed his back.

"Don't get up yet, Gabriel. We're okay right now."

"We won't be okay until we're away from here, Christy. I'm not going to risk losing you and our baby when we have another option. I'll get Jonah and Reba to get everyone from the church to start packing our things." He stood slowly and pressed a hand against his side. "Time to walk."

Christy expected the nurses would put a stop to Gabe pushing himself, but they encouraged him as did the doctor. They only stopped him the first time to bring him shoes. The educator returned to stress that he should never go barefoot even in their own home. They were given a book on foot care.

Christy kept her mouth shut and walked. She was reassured when the oxygen measurements in Gabe's blood rose steadily. By evening, he was able to dispense with the supplemental oxygen completely. The nurses removed the IV fluid, leaving the access device in his arm. He spent the afternoon using his laptop to complete lesson plans for the rest of the summer and his survey for the park service. At ten o'clock that night, Christy took the computer away from him.

"Go to sleep, Gabriel. You can't get everything done in one day."

"It's a nesting urge. You'll do it later. I'm doing it now." Christy turned off the lights and pushed the recliner close to the bed so she could hold his hand. A nurse came in and turned on the lights again. She checked Gabriel's vital signs and then his blood sugar. The reading was 188 mg%.

"You'll need a shot of insulin," she said. "I know you're new to this. 140 mg% is the top of normal for bedtime. We want to keep you normal so you won't have any risk of infection. Your immune system doesn't work well if your sugar is over 140 mg%. You'll also heal much faster if you're in the normal range. The new medicine you're getting with breakfast will probably get your sugar down without the shots. I'll be right back." Christy couldn't think of what to say to encourage Gabriel. He encouraged her.

"It's all right," Gabriel said. "I'm not afraid of diabetes now, Christy. I'm not afraid of anything I have the power to control. They sent a diabetes specialist, and he talked to me a long time. He's starting me on two new medications. One of them was that pill Bodine talked about. It's the one he called Avandia that makes your body more sensitive to insulin."

He pointed to a stack of pamphlets. On top was a brochure on Avandia. It showed a man saying, "I'm stronger than diabetes."

"I like that attitude. Forty years from now, you and I will be telling people that living with diabetes can be done and how to do it."

He was silent as the nurse returned and gave him the syringe. It was the first shot Gabe had ever given himself, and he hesitated for several seconds. When the nurse turned off the light and left them alone, Gabriel took Christy's hand. "I don't like needles either, but they don't seem to think I'll need the insulin very long.

"The medication they're starting with breakfast is called Starlix. It tells my body to make insulin just when I eat. Apparently my body can't make insulin for about thirty minutes after I finish eating. That lets my blood sugar go up and then I have to make twice as much insulin to bring it down. Starlix is the only medicine for increasing how much insulin I make that will work in the first thirty minutes after I eat and then wear off.

"The diabetes specialist said I'd probably need Starlix with every meal until I've healed and then I can just use it with supper or when my sugar goes up from eating wrong or being sick. I never thought I'd like the idea of multiple pills, but it's obvious that lifestyle and diet were too little and too late. I'd sure rather take the pills than carry insulin around."

"Why won't the Avandia do it alone?" Christy asked. "Why can't you take that metformin medicine like Mr. Bodine?"

"They said metformin doesn't work as well in people who aren't overweight. The endocrinologist says Avandia will probably control my sugar without any help in a few months. It makes me more sensitive to insulin at first. Then it starts to let the insulin making cells recover. That takes six months to a year. I might need insulin when I'm stressed until then, but I know how to give it. I won't do like my mother did."

"Did the shot hurt?" she asked.

"No," he said. "It's just the thought of it. I don't want to have to carry syringes and insulin unless I have to."

"I gave myself a shot today," Christy said proudly. "The educator taught me. She said it doesn't hurt as much when you don't bunch up your skin and when you don't use alcohol. She says we won't have to use alcohol when we're at home."

"That's different than when they taught me how to give it to my mother." Gabe shrugged. "I guess they change techniques when they find something better. When I took the shot just now, I thought about the baby. I can't tell you how much easier that will make everything else. When I was a kid, I always told myself I'd have a big family so my kids would never have to feel alone. When I never met anyone that made me feel the way you make me feel, I didn't think I'd ever have a family. I was serious on our wedding night when I said I hoped we were making a baby. I kept thinking about it that night when I was holding you. Are you happy about being pregnant?"

"I'm really happy about it. I was just nervous about telling you because of everything else that's happened to us. We haven't had a chance to talk about having kids. When you were unconscious, I didn't know it at first, and I told you that I had always wanted to have three or four kids and a house with a big yard and a garden." He was silent for so long Christy thought he was sleeping. His next words surprised her.

"I remember losing my family, Christy. I know that no matter what happens after that, it changes a child's life forever. We can risk our lives, but we have to focus our lives on taking care of this baby. We have to get away from here and start a new life together. You think I'm leaving here for you. Don't. In some ways, you'll be leaving here for me."

Christy slid the recliner forward and moved to sit beside him on the bed. When even that wasn't close enough, she lay down on the edge of the hospital bed beside him and put her arm across his chest very carefully.

"Wherever you go, I will go, Gabriel. Wherever you lodge, I will lodge. Your people will be my people, and your God will be my God. Wherever you die is where I will die, and I'll be buried beside you. The Lord do so to me and more also if ought but death part you and me."

She smiled up at him in the darkness. "We're just going to follow the cloud and see where God takes us."

Gabriel turned slowly to face her and pressed his hand against her abdomen.

"I always heard people say that out of every evil comes some good. That's us, Christy, and this baby."

"I'll let you name the baby if it's a boy, but if we have a little girl, I'm naming her Deborah."

"I was thinking the same thing." He kissed her forehead and closed his eyes. Christy lay beside him until she was sure he was sleeping and then returned to the recliner to keep watch over him. They were a long way from Cherokee before Christy felt safe enough to stop guarding her husband.

CHAPTER 24

It was a bright summer day in central Florida, and an art show was going full blast in the town square of Bakersfield. Several of the artists were working on new paintings in hopes of drawing attention to their work. One of the artists who was painting was already being watched by a New York art dealer and the president of the local art guild.

"That's Evie," the guild president said. "She's the most talented artist we have here."

"Evie Strongheart?" the dealer asked. "She doesn't look like the name." Evie Strongheart was very fair skinned and had long french-braided red hair.

"That's her husband on the blanket with the two babies. He's a Seminole. I guess he inspires her work. She's studying at the college. He teaches there."

The art dealer looked at the tall dark-skinned man and the two dark-haired toddlers on the blanket behind Evie Strongheart. Evie's husband was undeniably a Native American. Their children had slightly lighter skin, but their hair was straight and black. They had their father's very dark, almond-shaped eyes.

Mr. Palmer shifted his attention back to the artist and the gorgeous oils she was displaying. She was working on a painting of two Indian children learning the grass dance. Beside her was an oil of a woman standing on a precipice and reaching for the sunrise as it rose over the trees. It was that painting that kept his attention.

"That's a masterpiece beside her. I'd like to meet Mrs. Strongheart. I think she has a great career ahead of her."

Adam Strongheart stood and walked over to put sunscreen on his wife's shoulders and neck. "You're getting skin the color of your hair, Red." She smiled and looked up at him.

"Are you sure you don't need some?" she teased. Her husband rubbed a streak of sunscreen down her nose in response.

"I think my tan's pretty well maxed out. Put some on your face."

"Evie," the art guild president called. Evie looked up as she capped the tube of sunscreen and smiled her greeting.

"Hi, Margaret. How are you?"

"I'm doing great. I have someone I'd like you to meet. This is Joseph Palmer. He has a gallery in New York, and he attends the shows when he hears of new talent. The word is getting out about your work, Evie. He came to see you." Evie looked surprised and glanced back at her husband as if for reassurance. Adam stepped up beside her as she extended her hand to the art dealer.

"I guess I'm surprised. It's nice to meet you, Mr. Palmer. This is my husband, Adam."

"It's a pleasure to meet both of you," Mr. Palmer said. "I saw one of your paintings, Mrs. Strongheart. It was bought by a New York resident who winters down here. She's quite a collector, and she called me to see it. It's an oil she said you called the Eagle Dance."

"I loved that one," Evie said. "I started planning it after I saw the dancers the first time."

"I'm interested in representing your work, Mrs. Strongheart. I'm sure these four would sell within a week. They have an usually poignant quality." He wiped his face. "I'm not accustomed to this Florida sun. Could we go over to the soda fountain and talk?"

Adam turned and called to a teenaged Native American girl, "Laura, can you watch the twins for a little while?"

"Sure, Dr. Strongheart," Laura said. "Do they need feeding?"

"Not for an hour or so," Adam replied. "There's a bottle of water in the diaper bag if they get thirsty." He took his wife's arm and gestured toward the soda fountain. "This heat does take some getting used to."

Evie was giddy when she emerged from the soda fountain an hour later. Adam had left the meeting early because the art show was ending. He was loading the paintings carefully while Laura walked the twins in their stroller.

"And?" he asked his wife.

"He's taking them. He wants to see everything I've got, and I get a five thousand dollar advance." Evie threw her arms around Adam's neck, and they held onto each other for several minutes despite being in front of the town. "I just can't believe it."

"I'm not a bit surprised," Adam said. "I've known how special you are for a long time. Just don't forget about the little people who love you when you're rich and famous." He kissed her and then said, "I guess I'll be building crates tonight."

"I hope you're just joking about the little people in my life. You know how I feel. I'll stay up tonight and help you build crates," she said as she ran her hands over his back. "And there will be serious rewards for crate building."

"All right! I work better with an incentive." He lifted the last painting into their van and left Evie to pack her supplies while he tucked their children in their car seats.

"Come on, Win. It's time to go home." He buckled his son in securely and then took Deborah from Laura's arms. His daughter was squealing and increased her pitch and volume as her father picked her up. "Okay, little bit, you're coming, too." He kissed her dark hair and buckled her into her car seat with difficulty as she clung to his shirt. He turned to pay Laura for her services and then said, "We're ready, Mama. Let's go."

The Stronghearts lived on an older street in a renovated house from the early 1900s. The yard was unusually big and filled with flowers. Everyone knew everyone else in Bakersfield, and all the neighbors were outside despite the heat. They waved at the Strongheart family as they pulled into their driveway. Their next door neighbor, Camille, called out from her porch.

"Did you sell any paintings, Evie?"

"Believe it or not, I did!" Evie exclaimed. "There was an art dealer from New York, and he wants to represent me. We're shipping four to his gallery tomorrow."

"Congratulations. To think I'll be able to say I knew you when." Camille smiled. "How does it feel to be married to a famous artist, Adam?"

"I'm relieved, Camille. Teachers don't make that much money, and we'll have two in college at the same time." He unbuckled each twin and handed Win to his wife. He carried his daughter to the front door and unlocked it. He disarmed the security system just inside the house with a series of letters and numbers. Having the elaborate system marked them as different from the other residents of the small town. It included motion detectors. No one in Bakersfield suspected that the Stronghearts were a part of the witness protection program and had not been named Adam and Evie at birth. They were simply known as another mixed race marriage in a town near the Seminole reservation. Dr. Strongheart was a respected assistant professor at the local college. He taught diving courses on a contract basis. Evie was a part-time college student and mother who was making a name for herself as an artist. They attended the reservation Christian church and participated in all the church activities. When Evie had given birth to their twins a month early in February of the previous year, the church members had come to help Adam take care of his family.

Inside the house, Adam and Evie were Gabriel and Christy Killian, but they had lived their new life long enough to call each other their new names with familiarity. Gabe took the twins to the kitchen and put them in their high chairs before returning to unload the car. Christy was cooking supper when he returned to the house and flipped on the security system again.

"It's still ninety-six degrees outside," Gabriel said. "Maybe we need to use that advance to build a swimming pool."

"The springs are fifteen miles away. I think that's a waste of water." She handed her husband a divided plate of baby food. "Give me a hand here, would you, Daddy? Win is playing patty cake with his peas."

Gabriel looked at the food and grimaced. "Can't say that I blame him. Come on, Win. Hold your nose and pretend this is good."

It would have been a usual Saturday night at the Strongheart house if not for the continued celebration about Christy's contract with the art dealer. She had to read the document three times before she allowed Gabe to lock it in the fireproof safe. They ate their salad supper after the twins finished eating. They gave their children baths, and each parent read a story and rocked a baby to sleep.

Gabriel went to the garage while Christy cleaned the kitchen and started a load of laundry. It was her quiet time of the day when she could think of her happy memories. Almost all her good memories were of her life with Gabriel Killian. She stood in the hallway and looked at the picture of their wedding. She couldn't keep from smiling when she thought of their weekend in Asheville. She walked two steps further and looked at the first pictures of the twins after their birth.

She and Gabriel had only been in Florida for two months when they had learned she was pregnant with twins. She had experienced terrible morning sickness and lost eight pounds. On their first prenatal visit she had measured bigger than the only possible dates of conception. A million terrible thoughts had run through her mind while she was waiting for the ultrasound. Gabriel had read her thoughts easily and said, "I know who this baby's father is, Christy. No measurements can change that."

Fifteen minutes later, an ultrasound had revealed two tiny heartbeats Christy was shaking uncontrollably when Gabriel's hands closed on her shoulders. "We've been doubly blessed, baby. It's just one more thing to thank God for." His response had made it easy to be joyful and not worry. She paused to look at a picture of Gabriel standing behind her with his hands resting on her belly. Her husband had treated her as if she were beautiful even when she had felt monstrously big. His expression in the photograph was one of complete happiness.

Gabriel Wind Strongheart and Deborah Claire Strong-heart had been born on Valentine's Day, five weeks early for a full-term pregnancy but only three weeks early for twins. The expectant father had been a nervous wreck while they were making the usual prenatal preparations. He had insisted that the witness protection program be involved in the hospital preregistration. They had new names, social security; numbers and birth dates, but neither of them wanted Christy's blood type listed. In the end, they had avoided the standard procedure only by having their religion listed as one which refused transfusions. Christy's obstetrician knew his patient was a part of the witness protection program and went along with the odd requests after a federal agent reaffirmed the seriousness of the Stronghearts' predicament.

Everything seemed perfectly ready for the births until the babies chose to make an early debut on the only day their father was teaching that week. Gabe had covered all his classes for the following week but was conducting an all day field lab on Valentine's Day. Christy suspected she was in labor when her backache became rhythmic. She expected labor to take hours so she walked and did her Lamaze breathing as the pain became more frequent and intense. She thought she would have plenty of time even when the contractions were five minutes apart.

At four o'clock in the afternoon, her water broke as she entered transitional labor. Then she knew she had made a dire mistake. She had left an urgent message for Gabe to call her not saying why and called Camille. Camille had been home and had called an ambulance. They didn't have time to clean up the residue of the impending births and left blood on the living room floor and an unlocked front door to greet the expectant father.

Their son, nicknamed Win, had been born in the ambulance and had screamed as loudly as the siren. Deborah had been breech and her delivery had occurred on the stretcher in the emergency room. She had required breathing help.

The hospital was small, and a twin birth was exciting. In the turmoil, no one remembered to call Adam Strongheart until he was between the college and home. That faux pas had caused the new father to have a major anxiety attack while trying to locate his wife. Christy liked to remember her husband's expression when the local federal agent had brought him to her hospital room.

By then she had their son in her arms. If she had ever needed any proof, she would have known she was loved body and soul just from Gabe's expression. She closed her eyes and felt his arms closing around her.

"Thank God you're all right. I've never been so scared in my life." She could feel him kissing her hair. "You and these babies mean everything to me."

Gabriel's love had carried her through the long wait for Divilbiss' trial. Her favorite picture was of Gabriel holding his newborn son. She kept trying to capture the rapture on her husband's face in a painting, but that level of joy and relief seemed somehow elusive outside of a photograph.

She walked to their bedroom and looked inside their cedar chest where the framed eagle feather lay wrapped in a blanket. She had never forgotten all the things Gabriel Killian had told her about his dreams. All those dreams were encompassed in the framed gift from the Cherokee tribal council. Christy held the frame over her heart and prayed for her husband to have his dreams back. She knew God had used Gabriel as an instrument to give her what she had dreamed of having.

It was almost ten o'clock when Christy checked the back door's lock and turned off the kitchen light. When she entered the garage, she found Gabriel had two crates completed and a third in progress.

"You should have been a carpenter, Adam Strongheart." He turned and swept her off her feet and into his arms. Christy gasped and then put her arms around his neck.

"I'm multi-talented with the right inspiration." He carried her into their bedroom and put her down on their bed. He kissed her deeply and then held up his keys. "I'll be back in thirty seconds. Don't go to sleep because I've got to collect for two out of four crates."

"We need to practice our jujitsu first," she said.

"Lots of pins. No blocking." She laughed and rolled over on her stomach as he hurried through the house.

Gabriel checked every lock and then returned to the back door to change shoes. He had been wearing running shoes and socks. He shook a pair of clogs to make sure nothing was in them and put them on. Learning to wear shoes constantly had been very difficult for Gabriel. It had been one of the hardest parts of living with diabetes, but he complied to the rule even though his foot sensation was completely normal. He had been taught that minor injuries to his feet could result in terrible infections because the feet were in a dirty environment.

He walked back through the house turning off lights. The bed was empty, and he whirled as the door swung closed behind him. Christy attacked him from his left side and pinned his arm. He flipped her with his right arm, but she jumped to her feet and resumed a sparing position. She kicked toward his chest, and he swept her other leg and then caught her before she could fall. They both fell across the bed, and instead of continuing to struggle, Christy pulled her husband into her arms. Their hands entwined as their lips met.

"You made that really easy," he whispered.

"Sometimes more is just more, Gabriel." She rested her cheek on his chest and listened to his heartbeat as her own pulse gradually slowed. "This day was perfect, and sometimes perfect still scares me." He cradled her face in his hands.

"God's just giving you back all the time Divilbiss took from you, Christy. You're using all the talents you were given, and this is your reward. Don't let the past spoil it for you."

"You always keep me in focus," she whispered and snuggled closer to sleep.

"I want you to do something for me," he said.

Christy sat up and looked down at him. "I would do anything for you."

"I want you to paint another self portrait like the one we're sending to New York. I want to keep it. I've always loved that painting."

"You never said anything before now." She caressed his face. "You're the only person on earth who understands how I felt when I was reaching for the sunrise." She bent down and kissed him. "You were my sunrise, Gabriel. I'll start that painting as soon as I finish the grass dance one."

"Christy, you were my sunrise. You still are every day." He pulled her back into his arms, and they slept holding each other.

CHAPTER 25

———————◖▬◗———————

Gabe was opening their Saturday mail early the next morning when Christy came to their bedroom bringing a tray with hot tea for both of them. He tossed her a small velour packet.

"Don't forget."

"You're a far cry from the guy who didn't care about contraception," she teased him as she took her birth control pill.

"That was before I figured the percentage of salary going for disposable diapers. I still like the idea of four kids but not all at once." He took the four pills he had been taking for the last two years. One was the Avandia, which had controlled his blood sugar so well that it seemed as if he didn't have diabetes. He had taken insulin for two weeks after his chest surgery and had only needed it a few times since then. He took Starlix whenever he was ill and whenever he was off his diet. Gabriel knew his normal blood sugars of 120 after meals didn't mean he wasn't diabetic.

The normal sugars were because he had been lucky enough to be diagnosed and treated early. Since he had followed his diet, he had never had any side effects from the drug and had lost another ten pounds while increasing his muscle mass. He had studied everything he could find on diabetes and understood that blood sugar was a very small part of type 2 diabetes. The fact that his body was resistant to insulin and required a large quantity of insulin to keep a normal sugar was the real problem. He had made every diet and exercise lifestyle change that his doctors had recommended, but he didn't put his trust in just the lifestyle change. He took Avandia to protect his ability to make insulin and because so many studies looked as if the drug could prevent heart disease. He also took aspirin, the statin cholesterol medicine and his blood pressure medicine.

He had been changed to a different kind of blood pressure medicine just after their arrival in Florida because he had developed the cough Mr. Bodine had warned them about. He was taking an angiotensin receptor blocking drug that also protected his heart and kidneys but didn't cause a cough. His blood pressure had only been over the normal range of 130/80 with stress, but his doctor had explained that stress induced blood pressure elevations increased the risk of heart attacks, strokes, Alzheimer's dementia, and kidney failure. Medical studies had proven that low blood pressures in people with no symptoms were not associated with problems.

After being increased to the maximal dose of angiotensin receptor blocker, Gabriel's blood pressure was usually 100/60, which his doctor pronounced as excellent. His tests of kidney function had been normal every year, and his HgbA,C test of blood sugar control was always 6% or less. The American Diabetes Association dictated guidelines for all diabetics. The recommendation was less than 7.0%.

Christy leaned over Gabriel's shoulder as he took a drink of his tea to wash down the pills and opened the next envelope. She knew the contents of the letter before he said a word just from seeing Gabriel's expression. The letter shattered the perfect day she had had as she held onto his shoulders and read it with him.

"The judge has denied their attorney's motion for a further continuance, and the case will go to trial on August 31. We will notify you of your mode of transportation a week prior to the trial and help with any arrangements necessary to safeguard your children in your absence."

"I'll ask for a leave of absence that week," Gabe said. He put his hand over Christy's reassuringly. "Divilbiss isn't going to do anything. They've had months to find us, and they haven't. This isn't like when you were in Cherokee, and they had a birth date to trace you. When you testify in court, it won't matter anymore."

"I know." She moved into his lap and pressed her face against his neck. "I just can't forget how close they came to killing you. I don't want you to go, Gabriel. I want you to stay here and take care of the babies. I can be Deborah and go with Hawkeye and the other agents."

"No." His tone was adamant, and his eyes riveted her. "When you're in that courtroom, I'm going to be there with you. You'll be able to look in my eyes, and you won't be afraid to put Divilbiss away forever. I'll be with you every step of the way, Christy. That's my job." He kissed her and then threw the letter into the trash with perfect aim.

"Get ready, Evie Strongheart. We're going to be late for church if we don't hurry."

The fear was still inside her as they drove to church and during the services and Sunday school class. She prayed so hard that her fingernails dug into her palms during communion. She felt as if she were failing God and her husband when she couldn't push the fear aside. Having so much more to lose made the threat of Divilbiss seem overpowering.

It was the day for the church's diabetes support group. There were fifty people with diabetes in the small congregation. Some had had the condition for more than ten years and had complications.

Gabriel had started the group soon after their arrival. That afternoon a newly diagnosed woman in her forties came to the meeting. She sat quietly to the side while the rest of the group reviewed sample menus and discussed the latest issue of the diabetes journal they all received. They were all testing their blood sugar when the new member spoke up for the first time.

"Why bother? We're going to die. Everybody in my family has died from diabetes. It's like a plague. I don't see any reason to waste the money and time in testing what my blood sugar is. I'm just living for the next life when God will heal me."

"You can't do that," Gabe said. "All of us have wanted to give up at some point, but we know we can't. It's wrong to focus on the next life when we're supposed to be examples in this life. Our bodies are a gift from God, and how we've treated them is what caused diabetes. It's our duty to take care of ourselves so we can be healthy enough to serve God."

"How do you know you won't die anyway?" the woman demanded.

"I don't," Gabriel said. "I just know I would rather live and die with courage than with cowardice. If I couldn't stand up and fight against being a diabetic statistic, I'd send a message that my God isn't strong enough to get me through this. I can't believe and be afraid."

His words made Christy realize how she would have to face Divilbiss. She knew it was her duty to believe God would get them past this adversity as He had all others. She left her fears in the church as they drove home. She walked into her home with a strong heart and a strong spirit.

Carlton Divilbiss's attorney was already frustrated and angry before meeting with his client. He didn't understand how much worse he could feel until after the meeting. Carlton Divilbiss was backed by several of his business associates, and he was very calm for a man who had already been indicted on multiple counts of murder. He was out on bail because his attorney had generated sympathy for his age with a lenient, liberal judge. Divilbiss gestured toward the only empty seat in the room and said, "Well?"

"There's no other appeal, Mr. Divilbiss. We go to trial in less than six weeks. The court date is August 31, and with the evidence they have, it's probably time to plea bargain."

Divilbiss shook his head. "No. It's time to get rid of the witness. We already took care of the woman I hired to kidnap her." The attorney shifted in his chair uncomfortably.

"Mr. Divilbiss, you won't be able to find Mrs. Killian, and when they bring her to court, the entire army may be accompanying her. The federal people want to win this case. They know how many people were sacrificed, and they intend to get you."

"Mrs. Killian is in Bakersfield, Florida," Divilbiss replied as he stood to unveil a new oil painting. "She painted this, and obviously her husband, Gabriel Killian, was her model. My daughter saw it in a gallery in New York. The agent was very happy to discuss his new client, Evie Strongheart. I've already investigated the Strongheart family. The husband, Adam, is a biology professor at the local college. He served in the Navy and teaches diving classes. His military record is sealed under classified status.

"Mrs. Strongheart is twenty-three, and she's an art major. She gave birth to twins last year. Her son's name is Gabriel. Her hospital record excluded her blood type specifically. This is a copy of her driver's license photograph. He shoved it across the desk beside an annual from Tucker College. Looks familiar to me."

"Mr. Divilbiss, I can't arrange for anything like this. I don't have your connections."

Divilbiss pushed two sheets of paper and a check across his desk. "Those are your connections, Mr. Harris. I want Mrs. Killian brought here unharmed, and then we'll wait until her husband comes to get her. It might be possible to get her to change her testimony with the right incentive."

The attorney looked at the papers and then the check. "I'll see what I can do."

"You know your way out." Divilbiss waited until Harris departed and then looked at his bodyguard. "I obtained a copy of Killian's hospital discharge. He has no left peripheral vision. I'm sure you can use that information."

"You want him alive, too?"

"At least until we have both of them. Besides, he has AB- blood." Divilbiss was laughing as he left the room.

Christy had learned to dive with her husband, and it was her favorite recreation. Since Gabe had been teaching several summer classes at the time of their anniversary, they celebrated their second anniversary the first week of August after final examinations had been given and graded. Their twins were in the capable hands of Lily, their surrogate grandmother from church. Adam and Evie left Bakersfield to become Gabriel and Christy for one day and night.

Central Florida is known for having fresh water springs associated with underwater caverns, and Gabe was exploring them and documenting the plant and animal life for the park service. He chose a very secluded spring for their vacation, and they left their car in the nearest town to hike to the spring. Each of them had about seventy-five pounds of gear because of their wet suits and tanks, but Gabriel shouldered two-thirds of it. The hike was only ten miles, and they had stayed in good shape in case they might need to take flight. It didn't seem to take much effort to leave civilization.

When they had made camp, it was still early in the day, and they suited up for the dive taking light sources to explore the cave. Christy had learned how to roll easily into the water while holding her mask, and she was first into the spring. Gabe came right behind her and took the lead in descending to the bottom of the spring. The water was clear all the way down despite the depth of more than a hundred feet, and the fish were abundant and curious. Christy was fascinated and swam in a circle to look at everything while Gabe took notes with a wax pencil and board attached to his belt.

After thirty minutes they rechecked their air supply and entered the cavern. It was beautiful and alien, and Christy could have stayed for hours. Gabe was marking their route and watching the time. After three hours in the water, he led her back to the surface, holding her arms as they resurfaced. When their heads broke the surface, Christy was smiling so much that she lost her mouthpiece.

"You're wonderful."

"You're just easy to please," he said. He directed her toward the water's edge, and they climbed out of the water together. They stripped off their wet suits and returned to their camp. As the sun was settling into the west, they ate and then swam again using snorkels. By sunset, Christy was tired and stretched out on her sleeping bag. Gabe lay down beside her and held her until the stars came out.

"I wish we could stay more than one night," Christy admitted. "I always worry about leaving the babies until I have their daddy all to myself."

"When all this garbage is over, we'll go away for a couple of days. I have a rich wife so we can afford it now.

Maybe we can take a weekend trip to the Caymans and dive down the wall."

"Do you think I'm ready for the Cayman Wall?" Christy asked.

"I think you're ready for anything," he said. He took her hand and slipped something cool over her finger. She looked down in the moonlight in surprise and saw a new ring in front of her wedding band. It was gold and set with a central diamond surrounded by four smaller stones. "The big one is for you, and the others are for our babies. Eventually I'll get up the courage to try for more if you promise I can be there when the next one is born."

She looked up in his eyes and forgot about everything except how lucky she was to have Gabriel Killian. "I love you so much," she whispered. "I'll never be able to thank God enough to sending you into my life."

His smile was brighter than the moon above them and filled her with breathless joy when they made love. He whispered against her ear, "You are my life, Christy."

CHAPTER 26

———————————◯———————————

They made it home for church that Sunday and prayed to get through the trial. Praying about the trial became a daily ritual for them. Two and a half weeks seemed a very short time to Christy, and yet she prayed for the agony of the wait to be over. The threat to her family seemed much greater because she knew what it was to grow up orphaned. She didn't feel she had the right to pray for her own safety, so privately she just prayed for Gabriel and their children to be kept safe.

Sunday night Gabriel found Christy sitting up after midnight wearing the stereo headphones while their son lay sleeping on her chest. She was staring into space. He bent down to kiss her neck and removed the headphones gently.

"Do you want me to put Win down?"

Christy nodded, but she relinquished her baby reluctantly. She was still sitting on the floor when her husband returned to the living room.

"You've got class tomorrow, baby," Gabe said as he sat down beside her. "You need to get some sleep." She pulled his arms around her, and he could instantly feel the tension in her body.

"I don't think I can sleep," she said.

"What are you thinking about?" Gabriel asked. He thought he knew what her answer would be.

"Win and Deborah," she said. "If anything happened to me, would you be able to take care of them?" The words were a dart of fear in Gabe's heart, and she could see his fear when he held her face in his hands.

"Why are you asking? If you've got some sort of bad feeling about the trial, you're not going."

"It's not like a premonition. I was just looking at the babies tonight and remembering my parents died when I was just a little older than they are. I don't really remember them, and now I don't even have pictures of them. I want our babies to know me."

"They're going to know you," Gabe said soothingly. "You're going to see them grow up and graduate and get married. When they're a little older, we'll give them at least one more sibling. You're going to have to put up with me for at least fifty years. Don't let these people terrorize you, Christy. That's what they want to do. The feds have a good case, and after the trial, Divilbiss won't be a threat to anyone anymore." He pulled her against him and caressed her hair. "You know I'm going to take care of you."

"I know you are. I guess I'm just dreading this so much that I'm making a bigger deal out of it than I should."

"You're too tired," he said. He stood and pulled her to her feet. "You're doing what I did when I let the fear of diabetes get into my head. Come say your prayers and get some sleep." He carried her to bed and held her until she could sleep. After she was asleep, Gabe couldn't put aside the anxiety she had transmitted to him. He was awake until just before dawn.

Mondays between semesters were days when Christy went to the Seminole guild shop to work and teach teenagers who were interested in painting. Gabe always kept the twins those days, taking them on adventures. Christy left early that morning promising to be home by four o'clock. The only difference that morning from many others was when Christy returned to the back yard and put her arms around Gabe's waist.

"Hey, are you already back?" he teased as he turned to kiss her.

"I couldn't stand to leave without telling you how much I love you." She stood on tiptoe and kissed him. "You three had better stay out of trouble while I'm gone."

"I love you, too, but I can't make any promises about staying out of trouble if you don't hurry back." He hesitated to release her. "Why don't we go with you, baby? We could wander around the reservation until you finish teaching."

"No. It's too many hours to wander around with the twins. I'll hurry." She kissed him again. "I love you, Gabriel."

Gabe followed her to the fence and watched as she drove away. Then, he returned to their kids and their toy cars. He loved every minute he spent with his children and devoted the morning to playing with them. When they tired of riding their toy cars, he filled their wading pool and watched them splash while teaching them Cherokee words and songs. They were growing up bilingual even though it presented a risk since they didn't speak the Seminole language. Two members of the Seminole tribal council were aware of Gabriel and Christy's situation. They were both law enforcement career officers. They had assisted the Stronghearts in being assimilated into an unfamiliar tribe and stood ready to field any questions. It was a compromise that allowed Gabe to get past the loss of his heritage.

At intervals, the twins climbed out of the pool and tackled their father, squealing with delight when he tossed them in the air. Gabriel was almost as wet as his children when they had been in the pool for an hour. He was tired from his sleepless night and was contemplating a cup of coffee when he was tackled by both twins and soaked.

"You guys have your mom's ESP. This is a cold shower equivalent, isn't it?"

"Shower," Deborah squealed with delight. Gabe pulled off his soaked tee shirt and draped it over his daughter provoking wild laughter. He was extricating her when he heard the front doorbell ringing. Camille came to her back porch to call him.

"Adam, there are some men at your front door."

"Thanks, Camille." Gabe draped his shirt over a lawn chair and took each twin by a hand. "Come on, babies. Let's see who's here." He had a sinking feeling that it would be federal agents, and when he looked out the peephole, he knew he was correct. Hawkeye was in front of two other officers.

"I wish I could say I'm glad to see you, Hawkeye," Gabe said as he unlocked the door.

"They've made you, Gabe," Hawkeye said as he pushed his way inside. "Someone put out a contract on Evie Strongheart, and they gave Bakersfield as the address. We have an undercover agent in the Mafia, and he got word to us last night. We have to get you out of here until the trial."

Gabe absorbed the words in a rush and then ran to the telephone with both twins clinging to him. His hands were unsteady as he dialed the guild number.

"Pearl, this is Adam. Can I talk to Evie?" His face was eloquent in communicating the answer he received to the agents. "If you see her, Pearl, tell her to call me and then make her wait for me. We've got an emergency at home." He hung up the telephone and turned to the agents.

"She left here two hours ago, and the guild is twenty minutes away." Deborah seemed to sense her father's feelings and started to cry. Gabe bent and pulled both twins into his arms. Terror for his wife made him a bewildered husband and father. "What should we do?"

"We're going to find her," Hawkeye replied with confidence he didn't feel. He dialed 911 and informed the operator, "This is Agent Parker of the FBI. I have an emergency, and I need central dispatch. We have a possible kidnapping involving a person in the witness protection program. Her name is Evie Strongheart, and she's driving a van."

He was silent and then said, "I see. We'll be right there." He hung up the telephone and said, "There's been an accident, Gabe. There's a van that crashed on the road to the reservation, and the wreckage is on fire. I'm going to go look at the occupant."

Gabe closed his eyes to pray and then said, "I have to come with you."

"Don't. The occupant is dead, Gabe. If it's her—"

"It can't be Christy," Gabriel retorted. "I'd know it if she were dead. That's what they want you to think." At the same time, he remembered Christy coming back to tell him she loved him. The image froze him.

Hawkeye started toward the door and gestured to the other agents. "Keep them in the central part of the house and get the police over here to keep the street blocked off. I'll be back."

The agents had to be impressed by Gabriel Killian over the two hours that followed. He fed his children and put them down for a nap. Then he sat and tried to read his Bible. He had been praying for a long time when they heard the car pull into the driveway. Hawkeye and Gabe reached the door at the same time. Hawkeye put two rings and a charred silver cross into Gabe's hand wordlessly.

"It's going to take dental records. Are those hers?"

Gabe looked at the jewelry as if it were not real. It was all the jewelry Christy wore because he had been afraid for her to wear his dog tags after they had entered the program.

"They look like Christy's, but she's not dead. I know she's not dead."

Deborah cried out from the nursery, and Gabriel could hear Christy saying, "If we have a little girl, I'm naming her Deborah." He broke down and wept even when he went to get their little girl. The twins had never seen their father cry and cried with him. It took a long time for Gabriel to control his grief. When his emotions were exhausted, a blessed numbness kept him moving to get their children to a safe place.

A female agent was summoned and packed the children's clothes and toys. Gabe managed to gather some of his clothes and his Seal gear. As he stood in their bedroom, Christy was everywhere.

"Don't take her," he prayed. "Please don't take Christy." He packed her bag and prayed she would need the clothes he was bringing. He took their fire- proof safe to have their important documents.

Gabriel and his children were taken from their home for safekeeping, leaving the town to talk about the witness protection program and how you never really knew who might be living next to you. Gabe couldn't look back or even think as they drove out of Florida and into the night.

In an unknown town in south Georgia, the agents stopped at a safe house. Gabriel called Jonah and Reba and told them he was coming home with Win and Deborah. He couldn't say Christy's name without losing control, but Jonah and Reba knew what must have happened from their son's voice.

"Let us meet you, Gabe," Reba pleaded. "You don't need to be alone."

"We'll be there tomorrow night," Gabe said tersely. "Pray, Reba. Help me pray." After his kids were sleeping, he lay awake and begged God to let Hawkeye be wrong.

The telephone rang at 6 A.M., and the agent sitting guard answered on the first ring and summoned the team leader tersely. "Hawkeye."

Hawkeye came from the next room while Gabe sat on the edge of his bed and held Christy's jewelry between his hands as he prayed. He heard Hawkeye say, "Okay, I'll get back with you. Yeah." He turned to Gabe and said, "The dental records don't match, Dr. Killian. It's not her."

Relief washed over Gabe and was followed by rage. He stood to meet Hawkeye. "They did this to get me there so maybe we need to give them their wish."

"Dr. Killian, you aren't a Seal anymore," Hawkeye said flatly. "You're a good diver and a great marksman but this is a big deal."

"I think I know that better than you do," Gabe said sharply. "I don't need your permission. Lead, follow, or arrest me. Those are your options." He was going to check on the twins and spun around as Hawkeye grasped his shoulder.

"Gabe, I know where you're coming from..."

"Really?" Gabe interrupted. "Did you grow up with your mother in prison because she kept her husband from killing you? I know what it is to be a victim and to wait for someone to help you until you know no one is ever going to help you. My wife is a victim, and I'm not waiting while you decide if it's politically correct to take care of these animals. Afterwards if you decide to prosecute me, I'll go quietly off to prison knowing my kids have their mother."

"What makes you think you have any chance at all? You might just make your kids into orphans."

Gabriel picked up his Bible and thrust it into Hawkeye's hands. "Read about David and Goliath. That's where I'm coming from. When you finish reading, I'd love to get my hands on some C-20."

"You don't ask for much, do you?" Hawkeye muttered.

Gabriel took his son and daughter to the kitchen and sat them at the table to feed them breakfast. While he was putting little pieces of fruit and cheese in front of them, he dialed Tracy Tolliver's number and left an urgent message on his friend's voice mail asking him to come to Cherokee.

CHAPTER 27

They drove through the day and into the night to reach Cherokee, North Carolina. Reba and Jonah were waiting up for them. They had seen Gabe's children only in pictures, but Reba was born to be a grandmother. The twins had known no strangers in the Seminole church and allowed her to hold them.

To Gabriel's surprise and relief, Tracy Tolliver was already there along with five other former Seals he had served with. Their support reinforced his belief that he could get Christy back. He left the federal agents to talk to his former comrades privately.

"What happened?" Tracy asked as they closed the door to the guest room.

"Christy's an artist," Gabriel said. "She's been doing sketches and paintings since we met. She's been involved with the artisan guild on the Seminole reservation, and people have been buying her work. An agent from New York gave her a contract to represent her work in his gallery. The federal people think the agent said too much about Evie Strongheart to the wrong people. Divilbiss is in the Mafia, and he has connections everywhere."

"She left home yesterday to go to the art guild, and someone kidnapped her. They put a woman who looked something like her into our car and set it on fire. All they could recover was Christy's jewelry and dental records. The records don't match. I'm sure Divilbiss has her, and he knows I'll be after him until the end of time or the end of my life. I think he wants me to come after her, and I don't intend to disappoint him. I could use some help."

Even Tracy looked dubious. "Windrunner," he began.

"I don't want that kind of help, Tracer," Gabe interrupted. "This is my problem. I want some C-20, some wires, a remote detonator and some auditory surveillance equipment. I could use a satellite photograph of the Divilbiss estate. If any or all of that is impossible, I'm still going. God is the only power that could stop me."

"Gabe, what you're proposing is illegal. Even if he's holding Christy, he can have you arrested or even shoot you for trespassing and probably get off."

"I think I can make him afraid to do either one of those options if I have the right equipment. Think about it. Let me know. I'm going to get ready tomorrow and go Thursday so I need to make other plans if you can't help me." He exhaled slowly. "I just appreciate the fact that you came and listened even if you can't do anything else."

Gabe left the room and entered the darkened bedroom where his children were sleeping. He tested his blood sugar and found it was almost 200 from the stress. Stress had run it up more consistently than illness or overeating, but he had almost never needed insulin. That night he knew he would because the stress wouldn't end until Christy was home. When his sugar went out of normal range, his pancreas stopped releasing insulin normally. It was something the doctor called glucose toxicity. He hadn't wanted to take that issue seriously.

Christy had argued with him when he had tried to ignore a 198 during a bout of stomach flu.

"If you ever stop taking care of yourself, I'll leave you," she had said. "I love you too much to watch you kill yourself." He remembered taking the shot without hesitation.

"Behind every compliant husband is a wife kicking his butt." She hadn't been amused. He had pulled her into his arms. "I love you too much to give you a reason to leave."

He took a five-unit injection of short acting insulin and put the bottle of Starlix in his pocket to use at his next meal. Then he sat on the bed thinking of Christy until he had to escape the confinement of the house. It was a moonless night with clouds rolling in from the west, and he went to sit in the woods just behind Jonah's house. He was watching the clouds and the stars but his mind was on Christy. Jonah came outside obviously looking for him.

"I'm back here."

Jonah nodded as he approached. "I should have remembered. I used to find you in the woods whenever you were troubled. Your children are beautiful, Gabriel."

"So is their mother." Gabe made no effort to hide his anguish from Jonah. "Even hiding and living so many lies, we've been happy. It's been the best part of my life being with her. I don't want Deborah and Win to grow up without her. I don't want to live the rest of my life without her."

"Why can't these agents get her back?" Jonah asked with a father's pain for his son. "It's their job to protect both of you."

"Too many rules to follow. I'm the only one who has a good reason to break them, and if I knew they'd kill me or send me to prison, I'd still have to go because I love my wife." He shook his head. "I never understood how my mother could have accepted what happened to her. Now I know. Even with prison, she got what she wanted. She saved me." He looked at Jonah.

"If I don't get back, will you and Reba take care of our children as long as you can? I want them to have the right priorities, and if they were adopted now, it might not be that way. I feel guilty even asking you. You've been my father since I was six years old, and you didn't have to take me. I know I didn't make it easy for either of you. I never did anything to deserve what you've already done for me, Jonah. I'm sorry for all the times I didn't tell you how much I love you and Reba and how sorry I am for all I put you through." Jonah embraced Gabe and held him.

"I love you, Gabriel, and the apologies aren't necessary. You're our son, and I know you've always given us your best." He nodded slowly as he looked into Gabe's eyes. "If we needed to take care of the twins, we would. In my heart, I know you'll come back. When a warrior has his priorities straight, he can't be defeated. You are a warrior. When I look at you now, I think of David and Goliath."

The analogy made Gabriel smile wanly. "That's what I told the agent when he told me I might make my kids into orphans."

"I don't believe that will happen," Jonah said. "You have the strong heart my father spoke of. He would be proud to know you have his name."

The words washed over Gabriel like an answered prayer. He knew they were a sign that he could save Christy. He had no reservations holding him back as he faced his next challenge.

Tracy came out with Hawkeye as Jonah and Gabe were walking toward the house. He stopped to block Gabe's path.

"Gabe, we've all been talking, and we think you're playing into their hands. They know everything about you and your weaknesses. They'll probably even plan

to attack you from your left because they know you've
lost your peripheral vision."

"You believe that's why I won't succeed," Gabriel
said simply. "Let me show you something about having
no peripheral vision." He reached to take the handker-
chief from Jonah's pocket and walked to the center of the
yard before tying it over his eyes. "Now I don't have any
vision, Tracer." He never went barefoot, but he pulled
off his shoes and socks before assuming a jujitsu stance.
"Come at me."

Tracy Tolliver was surprised, but he assumed a similar posture. When he moved toward Gabe, his friend
easily countered every move without being able to see.
After a few minutes of sparring, Gabriel moved to attack
Tracy. He flipped his friend twice and finally stopped in a
kick with his foot inches from Tracy's throat. He stepped
back, bowed, and removed his blindfold.

"If you can feel it and hear it, you don't need to see
an attack to counter it," Gabriel said defiantly. "The Navy
said I couldn't compensate for no peripheral vision. That
doesn't mean it's true. We did the impossible for seven
years, Tracy. I never had a reason as good as the reason
I have now."

Tracy looked back at Hawkeye and then said, "I need
to make a few calls."

The twins came crawling and crying for their father
and mother as Gabriel returned to the house. Gabriel
gathered them into his arms and took them for their
baths and bed. He rocked them to sleep with one in each
arm, and Reba helped him put them down. Gabriel stood
by the bed for a long time and then bent to kiss both of
them. "There are so many things I want to tell them," he
agonized. "I want them to remember how much I loved
them." Reba put her arms around him.

"God will help you come home, Gabriel. He'll tell
you what to do. Make yourself listen."

"I am listening, Reba. I believe I'm doing the right thing. Keep praying for me. I know God may have another plan for me. I can accept that if Christy and our children are all right."

Tracy closed the door to his room in the hotel suite and spoke quietly into the phone.

"We all feel the same way, sir. We'll all have to resign and get into it with Killian if you don't give us some leeway. I guarantee we won't do anything to disgrace the uniform. Killian is taking all the risk." He smiled as he listened to the answer on the phone and then hung up the receiver.

"We're a go," he said to the other men. "Head out in the morning and get the supplies. They'll be delivered to the recruiting station in Knoxville by courier in the morning." He dialed the phone and when Gabe answered he said, "We're with you, Windrunner. I'll be back at seven to run through the plan. They're sending me an e-mail on the layout of Divilbiss' estate."

"Thanks, Tracer," Gabriel said. "Thank God," he whispered as he hung up the phone.

Job knocked on the door tentatively and then entered when Gabe said, "Come in."

He put his hand on Gabe's shoulder. "Mom called me and told me what happened."

Gabe turned and stood to put his hands on Job's shoulders. Seeing his cousin was a much needed moment of happy reunion. He was surprised by how mature Job looked. Long scars down both sides of Job's neck were reminders of the injuries he had suffered but so was his expression. The happy-go-lucky kid who had lived with Gabe was a man.

"It's so good to see you again, Job. I hope you got my letter."

"I did. It kept me going until I could get past everything that happened. I still have it in my Bible. Did Dad tell you I'm at the Bible College? I'll graduate in June."

"No," Gabriel said as he looked at Job in a different light. "But I know you're making the right decision just from your eyes."

"Are you going to try and get Christy back?" Job asked intently. "I want to help you if you are."

Gabriel put his hands on Job's shoulders again and took a long moment to gather his emotions. "I need you to be here with my kids, Job. I've asked your mom and dad to take care of them if I don't succeed, but I know it would be a big burden. If you're here, I won't have to worry about them. They mean so much more to me than my life."

Job embraced Gabriel. "I'm going to be praying the whole time you're gone, Gabe. I promise I'll be here for your kids for as long as you need me to be."

Several hundred miles away, Christy Killian was re-leased into a windowless room and faced her real captor for the first time. Divilbiss remained in the shadows with two bodyguards in front of him as he surveyed the small slender young wife and mother.

"You've been a tremendous amount of trouble, Mrs. Killian. But then again, your husband has been even more trouble. I don't like people who make me look like a fool, and he has. For now, you're going to stay alive because we both know Dr. Killian will try to get you out. I expect him to come by Thursday night at the latest." He nodded to a guard. "Give her food and water. Then I want her sedated." He pushed past the guards and walked over to finger Christy's long red hair. "For now, I'm leaving your children out of this, Mrs. Killian. If you fight me, I can take them. Since you and Dr. Killian both have the blood type I favor, your twins might make quite a few units of clotting factor."

Christy lost control of her ragged emotions and struck Carlton Divilbiss with such frenzied strength that it took both guards to pull her away. Divilbiss stood and wiped the blood from his lip with rage.

"Get me some clotting factor. Tie up that little slut and keep her tied. She can have water and nothing else. I don't want her too dehydrated to donate."

The guards gave Christy water and then tied her hands and feet, leaving her lying in the corner. She prayed for her husband and children all night

CHAPTER 28

Gabriel had gone over every detail of the Divilbiss estate until he could close his eyes and see the layout in his mind. He didn't expect the federal agents to come with him, but Wednesday night Hawkeye came to him and volunteered his assistance.

"You have to make this good, Dr. Killian. I don't want to have to arrest you."

"It's better than good," Tracy answered for Gabe.

"The only thing I can be charged with is breaking into his house," Gabe said. "I won't be using enough explosive to leave a detectable trace. If you have to arrest me for breaking and entering, I'm willing to bet I'll get off on probation. I'm not taking a weapon."

Hawkeye extended a bag containing a semiautomatic handgun. "Take this. It was seized during a drug bust so if you wear gloves, they can't prove you brought it into the house. We didn't change the registration yet, and it could be fun if we arrested Divilbiss in possession of this particular weapon."

Gabe nodded and put it with his gear. "Just get Christy out, Hawkeye. My kids need their mother. I'll get her to the fence no matter what it takes. If you can take her from there, I'm not worried about succeeding."

The hardest part was leaving his children. Gabriel spent every second with them on Wednesday until he put them to bed. Then he went running without permission from the federal agents and without telling his friends or family. He ran to the cemetery and found his mother's grave, though he hadn't been there in a very long time. The tombstone read Raynelle Windrunner Killian because she had legally changed her name back to Gabriel's father's name before her death. Gabriel knelt beside the grave and put his hands on the tombstone. He knew his mother's soul wasn't in the lonely plot, but he felt somehow closer to her there.

"I'm sorry, Mom," he said. "I couldn't understand why you lived your life the way you did, but now I do. I hope you know I'm sorry for being angry. I still love you, Mom. I always did." He said a prayer before leaving the grave. As he ran back to Jonah's house, he felt as if he were being strengthened for the battle ahead of him.

The team used a panel van painted with a roofing company logo and drove to the river that flowed through the Divilbiss estate at dusk, and then Gabe began the laborious task of applying all the extra equipment he had requested. He was surprised when he saw the other ex-Seals suiting up to join him.

"You guys don't have to go with me," Gabriel said.

"We have a lot of time invested in this operation," Tracy said. "We want to make sure it flies."

"Just get out when I get inside," Gabriel warned them. "I don't want anyone taking a risk except me. If they just get me, they'll think they have it made."

Tracy pulled Hawkeye aside as two of the other men checked Gabe's equipment and secured it under his wet suit.

"You know what's going to happen?" Tracy asked the federal agent.

"You know it has to look like an accident or Gabe will have to take the blame," Hawkeye warned.

"Unless you bring in specialists, it's going to look like a really unfortunate accident," Tracy assured him. "Gabe doesn't even know because he probably wouldn't go along with it. And you can always give him a lie detector test because he'll pass when he says he doesn't know anything about the accident."

"He's almost too honest," Hawkeye observed. "Sometimes any form of justice is a beautiful thing. All the kids in the quarry lake were under twenty, and they all died of exsanguination. The girl they killed in Florida was seventeen years old. Divilbiss is a vampire in every sense of the word. He deserves a stake through his heart, but this is the next best thing."

The divers hit the water at eight o'clock and began a four-mile swim in the deep current. They were swimming with the river's flow and using snorkels only. Gabriel was on the point during the entire swim.

They crawled out of the water and into the dark night at 9 P.M.. They waited for the spotlights to pass over them before crawling to the fence. Gabe took the small package of explosives and cut through the wire enclosure beside a large oak tree. He crawled through the shadows until he reached a pool house with its own propane tank to power the pool heater. He applied C-20 to the line leading from the tank to the pool in a thin almost indiscernible layer and attached a remote detonator.

When Gabriel left the pool area to reach the house, two of the other men moved in behind him and disabled the security system on one of the basement windows. Lights played around the perimeter before and after their passage, never seeing the hole Gabe had made in the chain-link fence.

Gabriel surveyed the entire house concealed in the shadows and then climbed a tree near a second story window and entered soundlessly. He knew he had tripped the alarm, but that was part of the plan. His only intention from that point forward was to reach the first floor study where Carlton Divilbiss would be. He was in the downstairs hallway when he felt an approach from behind him.

"Stop where you are and keep your hands where I can see them."

"I came to see Mr. Divilbiss," Gabriel said calmly as he raised his hands.

"I'm sure he wants to see you," the guard said. He took the gun from Gabe's hand and shoved his gun into Gabriel's back. "You're in the right hallway. Just open the next door and go inside. He's waiting for you."

Gabriel opened the door and entered the room as directed. There were three men seated and three other guards within the room. Divilbiss was a small gray-haired man with black eyes. He was seated at the desk and smiled as Gabe was pushed toward him.

"Dr. Killian, I presume," Divilbiss said derisively.

"Mr. Divilbiss, you have my wife," Gabe said calmly. "I've come to get her back." Divilbiss laughed.

"You're very confident for a man with four guns aimed at him. Bring Mrs. Killian, Jack."

Gabriel kept his eyes on Carlton Divilbiss as he felt the guard to his left step into the next room. Several minutes later he returned with Christy. She was obviously shaken and bruised, but Gabriel was so relieved at seeing her alive that he could hardly keep his eyes off her. His eyes told her to stay out of what was to come, and he was sure she understood. His expression calmed his wife despite their situation because she could see his camouflage had become war paint for that night. She was absolutely sure he was going to defeat Divilbiss. With her eyes constantly on Gabriel, she prayed.

Divilbiss pulled on a pair of latex gloves and picked up Gabe's gun. He seemed to aim it at Christy impassively. Before Gabriel could realize what was going to happen, Divilbiss had fired the gun and killed the guard standing beside Christy. Divilbiss put the gun down on his desk.

"Now we negotiate, Mrs. Killian. Your husband just broke into my house and killed my employee. I have numerous witnesses and a weapon with his fingerprints on it. If you allow us to videotape you stating that you made up the story about the blood farm, we won't report this murder. We will keep this gun, which I'm sure is registered to your husband, as an insurance policy. It will be a reminder to you of the testimony you've given here. You and Dr. Killian can go home and go about your lives without fear of reprisal."

"What if she tells you she won't?" Gabe asked. "You killed a lot of innocent people, Mr. Divilbiss. Seeing you prosecuted means a lot to me. I might be willing to be blamed for his death even though you pulled the trigger. I might be willing to take an insanity plea based on what you've done to my wife and my family."

"That would be a terrible mistake, Dr. Killian," Divilbiss said. "I can kill both of you tonight as easily as I killed him. With the only witness to my blood letting gone, they can't prosecute me at all. Oh, you didn't know we already took care of the woman I hired to kidnap your wife. She didn't find federal protection to be adequate either." He smiled at Gabe.

"I think of our little blood harvest as a sort of manifest destiny. My family and I are much more valuable to society than the potential for contributions from those college students. I think they donated their lives to our very worthy cause." Divilbiss expected to see Gabriel Killian's face reflect his helpless situation, but Gabe's expression never changed.

"I'll bet it's going to be very unpleasant for you to know everything you've just said is on tape in a van outside of this estate." Gabe raised his hand slowly and unzipped the top of his wet suit to display two wires. It won't really matter what you do to us because we have your taped confession, Mr. Divilbiss. They accept taped confessions in court, you know." He unzipped the suit a little further as Divilbiss looked at the guard to his left.

"You might want to tell him not to hit me. You know I don't see to the left and, of course, I knew you'd know so I brought my own insurance policy." He lowered the zipper to his waist revealing six white tubes wired to his body. All of the men stepped away from him.

"I don't suppose you looked into my Navy career, did you? My particular specialty was explosives. I just love to blow things up, and I got to do it a lot. These little tubes contain a substance called C-20. It makes dynamite look like a firecracker, and it can be detonated by remote control like this." He pressed his wet suit pocket and the house shook as the propane tank by the pool exploded. The flames illuminated the yard outside the study windows, and debris rained on the windows.

"That was one inch of C-20. These tubes on my chest are wired to go off if I fall down or if they get bumped. There's enough explosive on my chest to kill you and level this house. It won't matter how much clotting factor you've managed to make if the biggest piece of you is a quarter of an inch.

"I have a Cherokee sense of justice. We call it the balance. You may kill me and my wife, but I'll kill you and everybody in this house. I'll bet most of your family is here, aren't they? My idea of manifest destiny, Mr. Divilbiss, is acting as God's tool to send you to justice. That may confuse you since you obviously don't believe in God. You believe you *are* God. When you learn that you're subject to a higher power, you won't have access to an appeal."

Divilbiss hesitated as he studied Gabriel's stony expression, and then he gestured for the guards to step even farther away. They holstered their guns without being ordered.

"I underestimated you, Dr. Killian," Divilbiss admitted. "I won't make that mistake again." He looked at the guards. "Stay out of his way and give them a clear path to the front door." Gabriel didn't move.

"Just so you know. C-20 has a two-hundred-yard range, Mr. Divilbiss. If I get shot on your front lawn, you and your family had better be out of this house because it won't be standing. You also need to wonder how much more I have planted around here. I chose to set off your security system after I set up the charge at the pool. There are people in the Middle East with much tighter security who couldn't keep me out and didn't know when I got in. I had plenty of time to wire this house." He looked at Christy and spoke to her in Cherokee. "Walk out in front of me." Christy nodded to let him know she understood. He looked at Divilbiss as he peeled a transparent glove off his right hand. He tucked it into his wet suit.

"You can keep the gun as a souvenir. It doesn't have my fingerprints on it, and the feds said they got it from a drug bust. Who knows? It might belong to some friends of yours."

Christy was praying as she walked over to Gabe and began walking toward the door. The guards followed them but stood well back as they reached the front door. Gabriel opened it with his left hand and propelled Christy forward gently. He spoke to her in Cherokee as they descended the stairs.

"Go to the left. Run into the trees."

They walked down the stairs slowly with Gabe keeping his body between Christy and the house at all times. He could almost feel the guards aiming at him and prayed his bluff would hold until he could get Christy away. He was sure they were going to shoot at him as soon as they thought he was far enough from the house for them to assure their safety. When the trees were ten yards away, he said, "Run."

They ran as fast as their strength would allow, and Gabe heard the gunshots begin as they reached the trees. He shoved Christy into the cover and dove into it behind her just as he felt the impact of a bullet against his right thigh. The bullet took him to the ground out of sight of the guards but with an impossible two-hundred yards between them and the fence. He was struggling to get up when Christy dragged him to his feet and put his arm over her shoulders.

"Why didn't it explode?" she panted.

"I was bluffing. Unfortunately, they may know that now." He was able to run unsteadily with her almost to the fence while the guards continued to pursue them. His leg hurt, but it carried his weight. Gabriel knew they couldn't both make it to the river. He pushed Christy through the opening as soon as they reached the fence. "Get into the river. Tracer's there."

"Not without you," she protested.

"Go!" he commanded and shoved her into rolling down the bank. "The babies need at least one of us." He turned and prepared to fight the two armed men to give Christy time to escape. Their only hesitance in shooting him was their lingering uncertainty about the plastic tubes on his chest. As they both raised their guns, the house behind them exploded with thunderous force and collapsed into an inferno. The aftershock knocked all three men to the ground, but Gabriel recovered first and scrambled through the fence to roll down the hill toward the river. After six years of being a civilian, the water still represented safety to him. He was able to get under the surface and out of range before the guards could pursue him. They gave up the chase as the last remnants of the Divilbiss estate continued to light up the night.

Gabriel swam underwater using his snorkel until growing weakness forced him to surface. He thought he had traveled a mile, but he was already disoriented from blood loss and pain, and he couldn't be certain. He knew his leg was bleeding heavily, and he came out of the water to avoid the risk of drowning as his strength flagged. He had intended to tourniquet his leg, but when he crawled onto the bank, he felt and heard the fracture move out of place. The pain in his thigh overwhelmed everything else and completely immobilized him. He couldn't try to stop his leg from bleeding or get up to look for his partners.

When the pain finally eased, he felt his level of consciousness begin slipping. He looked downstream at the glow of the fire as he said a prayer for Christy and his children. He knew he was probably going to bleed to death before anyone could help him. He crawled toward the water knowing it would be better to drown and let the current carry his body far from the Divilbiss estate than it would for him to be found so near the ruins of the house. Before he could reach the edge, Christy grasped his arm. He tried to pull away until he recognized her in the darkness. That movement brought a fresh onslaught of pain that made him writhe.

"Where are you hurt?" she whispered anxiously.

"My leg," he said through clenched teeth. "Get away, Christy. They may still come after us."

Christy ignored her husband's request and pulled one of the plastic tubes free from his chest. She tore the wires loose and used them as a tourniquet around Gabriel's thigh. Even in the darkness she could see it was bleeding heavily. He groaned audibly as she pulled the wires as tight as her strength would allow.

"Don't leave anything they could connect to us," he gasped.

"I won't." Christy tucked the tubes into her pants pocket and took Gabe's hand. "We've got to get into the water. They won't be able to find us if we're in the water. I'm not leaving you, Gabriel, so if you want me to go, you're coming too."

He rolled into the water behind his wife to get her to safety. He would have submerged if not for Christy. His leg couldn't hold him even with the water bearing part of his weight, and he couldn't suppress the audible expression of his pain when he slipped. Christy supported his weight completely until they were four feet from shore where she could still wade against the current and pull him along with her. She supported her husband despite the fact that she weighed 110 pounds to Gabriel's 170 pounds. She wound her arms tightly around his chest, and that hold kept her from losing him when he was too weak to stay afloat. Above them a storm broke with thunder, lightning, and then a deluge giving them further insurance against pursuit.

Tracy and the other ex-Seals were in the water looking for them. They had heard and recorded the entire encounter in the Divilbiss mansion, but they had also heard the gunshots. They hoped Christy and Gabe were in the river but had no way to know for sure until they saw Christy with their night vision goggles. She was obviously struggling to hold Gabe's weight in the current. When he saw Gabe wasn't moving, Tracy crossed the distance between them like an Olympic swimmer. He shouldered Gabe's weight easily and carried him across the half mile to the van.

Gabe dimly felt himself being carried to the van, but the pain from being jarred made him regain consciousness as he was shoved inside. Tracy slammed the cargo door shut and jumped into the driver's seat to gun the engine. As they sped down the dirt road, the other former Seals removed Gabe's wet suit as carefully as they could. They still elicited enough pain to make him cry out. When the wound was completely revealed, the amount of blood was frightening. Jimmy pressed a gauze pad against the entrance and exit wounds.

"God help me," Gabriel gasped. Christy knelt beside him and lifted his head into her lap. She put her hands on his face and rubbed his temples in an effort to distract him. The tension in his body told her she was not being successful.

Rick had been a medic, and he broke open a first aid kit hurriedly.

"Hang on, Windrunner. They didn't equip this kit with any pain medicine. This is going to hurt like the devil, but I have to do it." He took Gabe's vital signs hurriedly and applied a tight pressure dressing to the bullet wound. Gabriel's fingers dug into the pieces of his wet suit, but he never made a sound. After Rick had splinted Gabe's leg, he placed an intravenous line in his arm and attached a bag of saline solution.

"Step on it, Tracy. He's still bleeding. I think they hit an artery. Jimmy, keep pressure over the bandage. Maybe that will slow the bleeding down."

Christy had been thinking of a leg wound as minimal compared to the chest wound Gabe had suffered two years earlier. Suddenly she knew the pain was the least of Gabe's problems.

"What can I do?" she asked Rick.

"He'll be okay," Rick reassured her. "He's been through worse than this. You can remove all the monitoring wires, Mrs. Killian. Use this cloth to get the camouflage off his face. We don't want anybody asking us why he's wearing them. We stretched a few laws to help Gabe get you."

"I don't know what you're talking about," Christy said as she met Rick's gaze.

"Good for you." He stripped the other transparent glove off Gabe's left hand. Then, he took the bag of IV fluid and began squeezing it to force fluids into Gabe even faster.

Christy peeled off the wires hurriedly and then wiped Gabriel's face. He was sweating so heavily that the towel was quickly soaked. His eyes were on Christy's face to keep his focus as he fought the pain. When she had wiped away every trace of the camouflage makeup, Christy held her husband's face between her hands.

"I love you, Gabriel," she whispered. "Stay with me."

"Call Jonah," he managed. "He and Reba have the babies. If I don't make it, they'll help you."

"You're going to make it," Christy insisted as she prayed for that outcome. "We need you, Gabriel. I can't live without you. You need to look into my eyes and focus on the babies."

"I'm hanging in there." He kept eye contact until the pain and his vision began fading simultaneously. She saw his lips move to tell her he loved her, but he couldn't voice the words.

The journey became much rougher as the van pulled off the road and stopped. The bouncing intensified Gabriel's suffering considerably and brought him back to awareness. His face contorted, and his breathing was audibly faster. Before anyone could protest, they heard the sirens of the county fire department and knew why they were hiding. They had to pull off twice more before they reached the interstate. Gabriel lost consciousness the second time, and pain no longer evoked any response from him. Rick couldn't hide his alarm when he rechecked his friend's vital signs. He and Jimmy applied a tight tourniquet above the wound and both men held pressure while another of the Seals kept the fluids running.

Even two tourniquets and direct pressure failed to stop Gabriel's leg from bleeding, and he was in deep shock when the former Seal team carried him into the nearest county emergency room. The ER doctor was quick to order red tag blood for an emergency transfusion and summoned air transport.

"We've got to get him out of here," he informed them. "He has a tear in a major artery, and he's bleeding to death. I've talked to the trauma team in Knoxville. If you sign consent now, they'll be ready to operate as soon as the helicopter lands. I have to tell you, he may lose his leg, Mrs. Strongheart. I had to cross clamp the two vessels to stop the bleeding, and he's not getting much blood into his lower leg. It all depends on whether they can repair the arterial damage fast enough. If we don't get him there fast, we could lose him."

Hawkeye took charge then leaving Christy to sign the consent forms. She was allowed to see her husband only for a few moments, and even with a large IV in his neck and two units of blood running, Gabriel was cold under her hands. He made no response to her touch. His leg was packed in ice.

Christy kissed his forehead and then leaned close to his ear. "We need you, Gabriel. Don't leave us. No one could ever take your place in our hearts or our lives." She kept her hand on his hand and prayed until the nurses made her leave. They gave her his jewelry while she was watching the trauma team load Gabriel into a rescue helicopter. The drive to follow him was long for all the people in the van.

CHAPTER 29

Christy spent a long night on her knees and was joined by Jonah before the surgeons came to talk to her. The surgery had taken more than eight hours, and the pink light of early morning was coming through the windows when Jonah touched her shoulder. She held her breath until she saw the surgeons' faces and then sat down in relief.

"Your husband is a very lucky man, Mrs. Strongheart. His thigh bone cut through his femoral artery. His femoral vein had already been injured by the bullet. I don't know why he didn't bleed to death or develop gangrene from having tourniquets on his leg for such a long time."

"We do," Jonah said quietly. The surgeon smiled.

"You're probably right. We took a vein graft from his lower leg and repaired the artery and the vein. Right now he has a strong pulse in his foot, but we won't know how badly the femoral nerve was damaged until he's awake. It appeared to be intact, but it runs with the artery and vein. His blood pressure was really low when we took him to surgery so he's been slow to wake up. We'll leave him in intensive care for the next twenty-four hours or so. This is Dr. Baker, the orthopedic surgeon. He can tell you about the fracture."

She scarcely heard the orthopedist's words, but after they had breakfast, Jonah made her understand the fracture had been repaired with metal plates to avoid any chance of the bone pieces moving. They were able to see Gabe for a few minutes after breakfast, but he was still sedated and on the ventilator. Christy and Jonah stood by the bed and said a long prayer of thanksgiving before going to the hotel next door so Christy could hold her babies. That reunion was tempered by knowing Gabe was still away from them, but she was able to sleep until the next visiting hours. Hawkeye met her in the hospital hallway.

"So far, so good. Since you have better support than I can give, I was thinking I could be doing something constructive like maybe giving Dr. Killian a homecoming surprise." He smiled at Christy making her think of him as a friend for the first time. "I had the feeling you might want to come back to North Carolina."

The answer was easy for Christy, and she signed the papers to restore their identities and to allow their belongings to be moved even before she went to see her husband again. To her relief, Gabe was off the ventilator, but he made very little response to her touch.

"Don't worry," the nurse reassured Christy. "He was in a lot of pain when he first woke up. He had some pain medicine just before visiting hours. If you're Christy, he was asking for you. Are you his wife? The record says your name is Evie."

"It's a long story," Christy conceded. "I'm his wife. Is his leg all right?"

"His pulses are great. So far, so good." She lifted the tucked-in sheet, revealing Gabe's foot. The color was reassuringly normal.

"What about the nerve damage?" Christy asked anxiously.

"He can move his foot so he has at least some neurological function," the nurse assured her. "We'll know more when he's more awake."

Christy kissed Gabe's forehead and stayed until she was told to leave. Then, she returned to their children and a vigil that was to last two days.

Gabriel heard the television in his hospital room as he returned to awareness, but the words seemed garbled for a long while. He felt someone check his neck and the bandages on his leg, but even that seemed surreal. Sometimes he felt pain in his leg, but most of the time he was aware only of being tired. He didn't know how much time had passed when Christy's voice pulled him back from unconsciousness.

"Wake up, Gabriel. You had surgery, but you're okay now."

He opened his eyes and smiled on seeing her red hair shining like a halo. It was a reassurance that he had not dreamed the successful rescue.

"I love you, Christy," he breathed.

She bent over him and kissed his forehead and then his lips. Her hair caressed him as she whispered, "I love you, Gabriel." She stroked his forehead gently. "What do you remember?" He had to think about his answer.

"Everything until the river." Gabriel shifted his position and caught his breath as pain stabbed his leg. Christy pushed the button on his pain medicine infusion to give him a dose. Several minutes passed before he could ask, "Where are we?"

"Mercy Trauma again. We've got to stop meeting like this."

"I'm all for that," he said. "When did we get here?"

"Three days ago." Christy caressed his face. "They brought you here in a helicopter. The bullet damaged a big blood vessel in your leg and fractured the bone in your thigh. When you had to keep bearing your weight on it, the bone moved and severed your femoral artery. You almost bled to death. They had to transfuse you with most of the AB- blood in Knoxville to get your blood count up to 25%. You've been in intensive care until now." Gabe shook his head.

"I can't remember anything after we went into the river."

"Hawkeye told the hospital you were doing some night diving and stumbled into the middle of a drug deal," Christy said. "When you were trying to get away, you were fired on. He'll be stressed out if you screw up his creative storytelling."

"Okay. I'll go along with anything he wants me to do now." He looked at her in relief. "Are you okay?" He put his hand on Christy's face tracing the bruise on her forehead. "I thought you were dead until the dental records didn't match. I've never prayed so hard in my life." He closed his eyes tightly. "Thank God you're back with us." There were tears in his eyes as he looked at her. "I love you so much, Christy."

"I don't think anyone could doubt that," she managed as tears ran down her cheeks. "I never dreamed you'd be able to do what you did."

"Faith can move mountains," Gabe said. His slurred speech told his wife he was going under the influence of the pain medicine. Christy's hand stroked his forehead until he slept again. He could hear conversation around him but couldn't decipher it until the next morning. The nurse awakened him then and took his vital signs.

"How are you feeling, Dr. Strongheart?"

"Better," Gabriel said as he scanned the room for Christy. He felt a moment of panic until he saw she was sleeping in the recliner.

"Do you need something for pain?" the nurse asked as she checked the bandages on his leg and neck.

"Maybe later." Gabriel pushed himself upright slowly and closed his eyes as a wave of dizziness swept over him. The pain in his leg was intense but tolerable. He was surprised to see the bandage covered all the area from his hip to his ankle. When his vision cleared, Tracy was at the door.

"No guts, no glory, Windrunner," Tracy commented. He came into the room and closed the door behind him. "We almost had to rename you Paleface after all the blood you lost."

"That's a horrible thought," Gabriel said with a smile. "You need to tell the other guys I'll spring for combat pay." Tracy sat down beside the bed and laughed.

"We wouldn't want you to waste future lunch money for your kids," Tracy said. His face sobered quickly as he continued, "I wish I could talk about what you did, Gabe. If we didn't have it all on tape, no one would ever believe us. I think you proved peripheral vision isn't all it's cracked up to be. If you ever decide you want to come back to the Navy, we could use that kind of thinking in intelligence."

"Thanks but no thanks, Tracer. If you'd made that offer two years ago, I'd have said yes in a minute. Now, it isn't important to me like it once was. There just aren't too many people I'm willing to risk my life for. A couple of friends and my family. I've got too much to live for to take a chance on losing it." He looked at Tracy as the memory of the explosion returned to him. "What happened to the house?"

"It had a central gas air-conditioning system, and the fire from the pool propane tank sparked the gas line. It was a horrible accident. The whole Divilbiss family was wiped out." Gabriel opened his mouth to question further and stopped because his friend's eyes communicated the real event.

"Thanks, Tracer. You'll never know how much I appreciate everything."

"This gets us even. The next time I'll have the chips to call in." Tracy nodded. "I've got to get back to Annapolis, but I had to see you first. We'll get together just for old times when you're up and around again." He put his hand on Gabe's arm. "Take care of your family, Gabe. Some of us wish we had what you've got."

Gabriel remembered seeing Tracy leave and then he slept again. The twelve o'clock news awakened him, and when he looked at the TV screen he' saw Hawkeye giving an interview to a local reporter.

"We've investigated the explosion site, and there's no evidence that this was anything other than an accident. There was a leak on the propane tank that fed the pool heater, and it was sparked and exploded when the heater clicked on. Then, the flames ignited the natural gas line that fed the heat pump. There weren't any survivors so we can't know beyond the physical evidence."

"Of course, Mr. Divilbiss had been accused of kidnapping local college students and keeping them hostage to use their blood in the so-called blood farm case. This case would have gone to trial in two weeks, but the victims' families will have to resign themselves to never knowing the truth. I'm Charlotte Bilbrey for channel nine news."

Gabriel reached out and put his hand on Christy's shoulder. At his touch she turned and moved to the edge of the bed very carefully. Her hands felt wonderfully cool on his face.

"I've really missed your company, Dr. Strongheart. I thought you were going to sleep forever." Her face clouded for a moment. "I was afraid I was going to lose you. All I could do was pray and cry."

"No more tears," he said. "It's over. He can't ever hurt us again."

"It's over because of you, Gabriel," she said.

"I can't take credit for it," Gabe said. "I kept praying, and then I knew what to do. When I can get on my knees,

I'll be thanking God for the rest of my life for letting it work."

Christy kissed his forehead and then his lips. "I've been thanking Him pretty constantly since they said you weren't going to die or lose your leg." She wiped her eyes. "Now all we have to do is figure out where we want to spend the rest of our lives."

"You choose," Gabriel replied. "When we get out of here, I'll have everything I want. I can be happy in any place where you and the twins are." He looked at her hand and smiled. Reba had obviously returned Christy's rings and cross to her. He glanced at his own left hand, seeing his wife had returned his ring.

"Everybody in Bakersfield knows we aren't Adam and Evie Strongheart now."

"Let's come back to Cherokee, Gabriel. I like Bakersfield, but Reba and Jonah are here, and family is the most important thing of all. I'm getting my dream. I'd like to see you have yours."

"You and the twins are my dream, Christy. Everything else we get is just a blessing." She moved closer to hold him very tightly, and she could feel that they were of one heart and one mind. When she looked in Gabe Killian's eyes, she couldn't feel any regrets for the arduous journey she had taken to find her home.

Gabriel was given crutches the next day and worked with physical therapy for the next three days. The orthopedist had a lengthy list of instructions before writing the discharge orders because the bullet had fractured Gabe's femur, the largest bone in the body, and the metal plates and screws were at high risk for infection because of his stint in the river afterwards and his diabetic condition. The later seemed the least of their worries. He had required insulin only twice in the intensive care unit. Even missing his Avandia dose for a few days hadn't made any difference because the effects were present

for months after stopping the drug. It was the first thing
Gabriel asked for on awakening.

A neurologist also came to check Gabriel's leg for
strength and sensation. He seemed surprised at his
findings and told them Gabe's femoral nerve seemed
remarkably intact.

"There has to be some damage, Dr. Strongheart, but
whatever it is will no doubt resolve in time. If you have
any trouble when you start weight bearing, we'll check
you again."

Gabriel went through all of medical procedures with
unusual patience until the last day because he was focused on getting out. Then, his only concern was Christy's
absence. She had gone ahead to Cherokee supposedly
to get Reba's spare room ready. By the second afternoon
without his wife, Gabe's patience was exhausted. He was
grateful for Hawkeye's offer of a ride back to Cherokee.
The agent picked him up in a new van bearing their
Florida plates.

"I guess you're telling me we don't need protection
any more," Gabriel observed as they drove out of the
parking lot.

"There's another car following us, but they're only
coming to give me a ride. The word from our Mafia connection is that no one is going to miss Divilbiss enough
to come asking questions. Since the destruction was so
complete, no one ever will be able to prove you were
there. I know you didn't set the main charges, and there
aren't any traces of C-20 left to implicate you or your
friends or me." Hawkeye smiled grimly. "There wasn't
a trial, but there was definitely punishment. Sometimes
punishment is enough." He glanced at Gabriel. "So what
will you do now?"

"The doctors say I'm going to be sitting around for
at least the next six weeks. It's too bad you have me as a
Seminole or I could get free care in Cherokee. I guess I'll
have to burn up the road to Asheville." He shrugged as

his eyes saw the dim blue line of the Smoky Mountains. "It will be good to come home even for a while."

"We can undo what we did, Gabe. You can be resurrected as Dr. Gabriel Killian."

"I'll have to talk to Christy," Gabriel replied slowly. "We'll have to make that decision together. She had just gotten her career as a artist going. I don't want her to lose out on that chance."

"We already talked to her agent," Hawkeye said. "He knows you're in the witness protection program, and it didn't bother him a bit." Hawkeye glanced at Gabriel again. "If it were your choice, where would you be?"

"Where Christy wants to be." Gabe smiled. "I love these mountains, but I love my family more. Right now, all I want to do is see my kids. There were a few minutes on that river bank when I thought I might not see them again in this life. I'm really glad God didn't ask me to make that sacrifice."

"I think you already proved what your family means to you. You know you could probably have a job with the agency if you wanted one." Gabe's face answered Hawkeye's offer.

"You don't need a biology teacher on your payroll, Hawkeye. Find somebody younger with nothing to lose. I've got a family to raise and all sorts of plans for my life's work." He sat back and focused on the mountains. "You make me nervous when you're this congenial. Are you sure you don't have an agenda?"

"I'm just enjoying being the good guy for once, Dr. Killian," the agent replied. "And I'm enjoying being a part of a happy ending. Sometimes breaking the rules can be very gratifying."

Gabriel was tired, but he kept his eyes on "the hills" all the way back to Cherokee. Because it was still summer, it was only evening when they drove into Qualla Boundary. He was startled from his reverie when the agent turned off Highway 441 onto the street where he had lived. Before he could ask the question, he saw a crowd of family and friends gathered in the front yard. Christy and Reba were at the forefront holding the twins.

"You said you wanted to be where Christy wanted to be," Hawkeye said. "She didn't even hesitate." The agent passed a bag to Gabriel as he stopped the car. "There's your new ID. All you need to do is paint Killian on the mailbox."

Job came to open the car door, but Gabe turned to shake Hawkeye's hand before reaching for his crutches.

"There were a few times when I wanted to knock you out, but you've been a friend a lot more than you were an enemy. Thank you."

"Good luck, Dr. Killian," Hawkeye smiled. "If you change your mind about that job..."

Gabriel shook his head and stood with Job's help. "Good luck to you, Hawkeye." Moments later he was embracing his wife and children. Hawkeye waited to leave until the Killians were surrounded by family and friends. He drove away feeling satisfied that his job had been well done. He would have liked to have seen Gabe's face when he saw his home restored to its former state. He had helped Christy hang a framed eagle feather over the fireplace but didn't ever learn of its significance.

Hawkeye didn't expect to return to Cherokee, but six months later he was in there again to watch the Killians renew their wedding vows. The ceremony was conducted like a Navy wedding with Gabe wearing his dress white uniform. Tracy Tolliver was there as best man. Jonah gave the bride away, and Job Killian performed the ceremony. At the party afterwards all of their friends came to celebrate the Killian's marriage. No one seemed happier than Jonah and Reba Killian as they held the twins, their first grandchildren, because they knew Christy and God had finally brought Gabriel Killian home.

Printed in the United States
22350LVS00002B/319-336